Counselling Skills for Health Professionals

OTHER BOOKS BY PHILIP BURNARD PUBLISHED BY STANLEY THORNES

- *Acquiring Interpersonal Skills: a Handbook of Experiential Learning for Health Professionals*, 2nd edition
- *Effective Communication Skills for Health Professions*, 2nd edition
- *Writing for Health Professionals: A Manual for Writers*, 2nd edition
- *Personal Computing for Health Professionals*

ABOUT THE AUTHOR

Philip Burnard is Professor and Vice Dean at the University of Wales College of Medicine, Cardiff, UK. He is also Honorary Lecturer at the Hogeschool Van Utrecht, Netherlands, and he has lectured in Finland, Sweden, Hong Kong, Brunei, Australia, China and the Caribbean. He is the author of 32 books on counselling, communication, ethics, research methods, writing, computing, supervision and mentoring, education and training and has published widely in journals in the UK, USA, Finland, Hong Kong, Romania, the Czech Republic and Italy. Professor Burnard's research interests include AIDS counselling, teaching and learning styles, experiential learning, self-disclosure and crosscultural views of mental health and mental illness. He is currently engaged in projects in Hong Kong, China and Thailand. In 1996 he was made a Fellow of the Florence Nightingale Foundation for his educational and overseas work. He was promoted to a Personal Chair at the University of Wales in 1998.

Counselling Skills for Health Professionals

Third edition

Philip Burnard PhD
University of Wales College of Medicine
Cardiff, UK

Stanley Thornes (Publishers) Ltd

First edition published in 1989
Second edition published in 1994 by Chapman & Hall
Third edition published in 1999 by:

Stanley Thornes (Publishers) Ltd
Ellenborough House
Wellington Street
Cheltenham
GL50 1YW
United Kingdom

99 00 01 02 03 / 10 9 8 7 6 5 4 3 2 1

A catalogue record for this book is available from the British Library

ISBN 0 7487 3976 9

Typeset by WestKey Ltd., Falmouth, Cornwall
Printed and bound in Great Britain by Martins The Printers Ltd., Berwick upon Tweed

CONTENTS

Acknowledgements

I am grateful to the many people who have played a part in the development of this book. Jo Campling was originally responsible for the first edition.

Thanks go to the team at Stanley Thornes who have always been supportive and helpful. I have learned a great deal from the people who have edited and subedited my books in this series.

Particular thanks goes to my personal assistant, Joy Slack, who has contributed so much to the preparation of this and other texts.

The author thanks the British Association for Counselling for their permission to reproduce their various codes of ethics and practice for counsellors, trainers and supervisors. It is acknowledged that permission was given on the condition that readers note that the BAC's codes of conduct are updated on a regular basis and that readers should check with the BAC in order to ascertain that the particular Code printed is the latest one available.

Finally, as ever, thanks to my wife, Sally, to my son, Aaron, and to my daughter, Rebecca. Sally has always been supportive. Aaron taught me how to use a computer and Becky cheers me up. Thanks.

INTRODUCTION

This is the third edition of a book that I hope continues to be of practical value. For counselling must always be that: practical. No amount of talking, on its own, can really make a difference if people do not end up doing something as a result of counselling. The practical thread remains an important one throughout this edition.

Counselling Skills for Health Professionals is not just a 'how to do it' book: people are probably too complicated for that approach to be of much use. Counselling is never simply a matter of learning a range of skills which you then apply in a range of settings. In the end, counselling is about facing the person in front of you, listening to them carefully and then supporting them as they work through their problems. For many problems, there are no easy answers and counselling doesn't offer any 'quick fixes'. It is essentially a supportive process. There are many things it cannot do. It cannot change certain social and political situations. It cannot cure diseases. On the other hand, what it can do is offer people more hope. Often, just the fact that there is someone who is prepared to hear your story and to listen to you is all that is needed. I remain convinced that the key issue in all types of counselling is the ability to listen. Some of the best counselling involves the counsellor remaining silent for a lot of the time. In the end, we all need to be listened to.

The basic structure of this book remains unchanged although many new sections, checklists and reports from the theory and research have been added. The first part of the book explores a range of theoretical issues: what counselling is, the issue of self-awareness in counselling and maps of the counselling process. The second part of the book considers specific counselling skills: listening and attending, counselling interventions, coping with feelings and support for the counsellor. I sense that there has been a subtle change in counselling theory away from an almost exclusively client-centred approach towards one that involves information giving as well as facilitation. I have explored some of these issues in relation to up-and-coming approaches such as the cognitive-behavioural approach.

The last part of the book focuses on practical methods of developing counselling skills and is addressed to three groups of people: those working on their own, those working in pairs and those learning counselling in small groups. Practical suggestions are made about how to set up and run counselling skills groups. The book then offers a range of counselling skills exercises that can be used by any of the aforementioned three groups of people. The emphasis, throughout, has been on keeping things simple without (I hope) glossing over the complexities of the human condition. For this is the paradox: that while simple counselling strategies often make a lot of difference, human beings continue to be as complex and varied as ever. The book closes with a bibliography of recommended reading and references.

I hope that the increasing call for health education and for self-direction in health care will mean that the skills explored in this book will be useful to a wide range of people, from the individual who wants to enhance his or her counselling skills to the lecturer or teacher who wants practical ideas about running counselling skills workshops. I know, too, that the book has been useful on some counselling certificate and diploma courses.

We all have problems in our lives and counselling offers one means of exploring and relieving some of them. While I don't believe that counselling is the answer to all problems, nor do I believe that counselling is something that should and can only be done by trained professionals. After all, we all counsel our friends and families on a daily basis. I do not believe, either, that there is any one right way to go about counselling. We must not overestimate the degree to which what we do affects other people. In the end, it is the person referred to as the client who makes a difference to his or her own life. In the end, the client sorts themselves out. I know, though, that careful and honest listening can make a difference. All health professionals can benefit from training themselves to become better listeners, to avoid rushing in to 'fix' things for other people, and from standing back to allow people to sort themselves out. This book is aimed at developing some of those essential skills. I hope it is readable and practical.

Philip Burnard
Caerphilly, Wales, UK

For Joy Slack, for her help on this and many other projects.

1 What is counselling?

It is difficult to avoid references to counselling these days. After disasters, after political upheavals, after any group of people has had to face a difficult situation, we are informed that the participants in those dramas were 'offered counselling'. We may question the timing. It is debatable whether a person 'needs counselling' directly following a dramatic event, at some time after it or at all. I suspect that there is a wide range of people from those at one end of the scale who benefit, considerably, from talking things through to others at the other end of the scale who prefer to work through their problems and reminiscences in private. At the outset, I would like to stress my belief that counselling is not necessarily for everyone and that, clearly, it would be bizarre and presumably unhelpful to foist counselling on those who do not want or need it. If we believe – as do many counsellors – that people differ from one another and that, in the end, they are the identifiers of their own solutions to their own problems, then it follows that counselling will suit and help some people and not others.

In a sense, we are all counsellors. Anyone who works in one of the health professions and comes into regular contact with people who are distressed in any way, whether psychologically, physically, spiritually or practically, offers counselling help. Counselling is something familiar to everyone. There need be no mystique about it. Nor should it be something that is reserved for a particular group of professionals who call themselves counsellors. As we shall see, it is useful to talk about *acting as a counsellor* and *using counselling skills*. Thus the discussion is already focused on familiar territory, although we can always get to know it better. The aim of this book is to explore some of the many facets of counselling and to encourage health professionals to identify ways in which their counselling skills may be improved. All skills are learned. This is true irrespective of any particular psychological point of view we hold. Whether we would call ourselves behaviourally, psychodynamically or humanistically oriented, there is little doubt that we learn and develop skills as we grow, train and live. It is difficult to argue otherwise and to say that we are born with counselling skills.

If it is true that we learn skills in this way, then it also follows that we can improve our interpersonal skills. This book focuses on that argument and is a practical guide to enable the already functioning health care counsellor to become better. The practical skills described in this book may be used in a variety of situations, from talking through a period of work-related stress with a friend to coping with a client in emotional crisis. The skills involved in these situations turn out to be remarkably similar. There are basic human skills that can be applied to almost all human situations. In the end, we are always working with another human being who is remarkably like ourselves underneath the skin.

There are also pitfalls to be avoided and these are discussed. Human problems are rarely profession specific. Whilst the doctor deals with aspects of the human situation in a different sort of way from how the physiotherapist would and the nurse is responsible for different aspects of care from the speech therapist, in the end, the difficulties that arise through the process of living turn out to be the domain of all health professionals. We all suffer from the same sorts of problems or, as Carl Rogers, founder of client-centred counselling, noted: 'What is most personal is most universal' (Rogers, 1967). The fact that we live at all gives us a clue to the sorts of problems that anyone can suffer and to how others overcome their problems. This is not to say that everyone perceives their problems in the same way but that suffering is universal. Anyone concerned for another person's health and well-being needs, necessarily, to be concerned for what may be called that person's *problems in living*. It is towards these problems in living that counselling is directed.

The *process* of counselling can be defined as the means by which one person helps another to clarify his or her life situation and to decide further lines of action. Lack of clarity often brings anxiety. We are frightened by what we do not know or understand. Such fear and lack of clarity often lead, in turn, to inaction. This is often true in health care settings. The patient or client who is suffering from chronic illness may find it difficult to plan ahead, often through fear born out of lack of information about their condition. The aim of counselling must be to free the person being counselled to live more fully and such fuller living comes through action. In the end, counselling must have a practical aim. It can never be 'only talk'. It must seek to empower the client to become confident enough to choose a particular course of action and see it through. In this sense, counselling is also a form of *befriending*, of supporting the other person. Again, such befriending is familiar to us all and is a vital part of any person's job in the health professions.

The nurse befriends the psychiatric patient when in the role of community psychiatric nurse. Social workers very clearly befriend the families with whom they work and GPs become a friend to many of their patients. It is clear that an immediate requirement of anyone who seeks to work as a counsellor is that they must like people. This concept of befriending is discussed further in Chapter 3, under the heading of the qualities of an effective counsellor.

Although a wide range of books describe various approaches to defining counselling, perhaps one of the most all-encompassing and exhaustive of definitions is that offered by Feltham and Dryden (1993). They suggest that counselling is:

> ***a principled relationship characterised by the application of one or more psychological theories and a recognised set of communication skills, modified by experience, intuition and other interpersonal factors, to clients' intimate concerns, problems or aspirations. Its predominant ethos is one of facilitation rather than of advice-giving or***

> *coercion. It may be of very brief or long duration, take place in an organisational or private practice setting and may or may not overlap with practical, medical and other matters of personal welfare. It is both a distinctive activity undertaken by people agreeing to occupy the roles of counsellor and client . . . and it is an emerging profession . . . It is a service sought by people in distress or in some degree of confusion who wish to discuss and resolve these in a relationship which is more disciplined and confidential than friendship, and perhaps less stigmatising than helping relationships offered in traditional medical or psychiatric settings.*

In this book, we will discuss each of the various issues that arise out of Feltham and Dryden's definition.

COUNSELLING OR COUNSELLING SKILLS?

This book is about counselling skills. It is not, necessarily, about the process of becoming a counsellor. What's the difference? Some people work as full- or part-time counsellors. Their job is to counsel other people and if they were asked what they did, they would say that they were a counsellor. Many other people use a range of skills associated with counselling in their everyday work as health professionals. Thus, a distinction can be made between *working as a counsellor* and *using counselling skills*. Not all health professionals who use counselling skills will work as counsellors although all counsellors will obviously use counselling skills. The prime aim of this book is to encourage those working as health care professionals to think about ways in which they can use counselling skills in their everyday practice. It is not assumed that everyone reading it will want to function, primarily, as a counsellor although, clearly, the book will have relevance to professional counsellors as well. Readers should also consult appendices 1 and 3 in order to consider the British Association for Counselling's definitions of counselling and counselling skills.

AN ACT OF FAITH

Counselling is also much more than just skills, processes and procedures. It is more, even, than words, plans and actions. It is also about faith. Whilst the efficacy of counselling, from the point of view of research, has not been established, those who practise it do so because they believe in other people and in the power of helping people to tell their stories. We counsel, I suspect, because we have faith in it.

> *And how shall we be able to administer help to others without the Faith of the Counsellors? (Halmos, 1965)*

Nor are we born equal. This is as much true of our personality structures as it is of any other social, physical or cultural variables. William James, one of the founding fathers of modern psychology, made this observation, which seems to sum up the vagaries of human nature:

> *Some persons are born with an inner constitution which is harmonious and well balanced from the outset. Their impulses are consistent with one another, their will follows without trouble the guidance of their intellect, their passions are not excessive and their lives are little haunted by regrets. But there are others whose existence is little more than a series of zigzags, as now one tendency and now another gets the upper hand. Their spirit wars with their flesh, they wish for incompatibles, wayward impulses interrupt their most deliberate plans, and their lives are one long drama of repentance and effort to repair misdemeanours and mistakes. (James, 1890)*

Fortunately or unfortunately, it is these differences which make us human. However, it also remains the case that, at some point, we need to undertake thorough 'outcome' studies to identify whether or not counselling really makes a difference to people in the long term. Whilst counselling has become a popular activity, there has been relatively little research undertaken to prove or disprove the ultimate value of it. One of the problems of such research is allowing for what are sometimes called 'confounding variables'. In the end, there are so many things that impinge on any particular person's life that it is probably impossible to say, one way or the other, that it was counselling that made the most importance difference to a difficult life situation. However, we live in a time when health care has to be shown to be cost effective. It cannot be long before those who encourage counsellors to use their skills or who buy the skills of counsellors for their health care programmes begin to demand proof of those counsellors' effectiveness.

THE WILL TO CHANGE

Perhaps one of the most important concepts in counselling, from the client's point of view, is the will to change. Sigmund Freud is often accredited with saying that the last thing a neurotic person wants to lose is their symptoms. So it can be with those who seek counselling. If counselling is to be effective, then the client has, to a greater or lesser extent, to *change*. Sometimes, people come to counselling expecting that either the counsellor will somehow change them or the process of counselling, itself, will change them. What has to happen, of course, is that the client has to change: nothing will come of counselling if the only change is the counselling itself. We might put it, oversimply, as follows: the client, during the process of counselling, needs to be able to identify:

- those things that they have to *do*;
- those things that they have to *stop doing*;
- those things that they need to *continue to do*;
- those things that they need to *accept*.

These points can become concrete aims in any counselling relationship. The counsellor can help the client to identify those things that he or she has to do, stop doing, continue to do or accept. It seems likely that almost all counselling involves a mix of these things. There is, perhaps, much truth in those old American saws: 'If it ain't broke, don't fix it' and 'If it works, do more of it'.

Also important is the *rate of change* or the slope at which change is introduced. Too much change too quickly is likely to overwhelm the client and force him or her to see a 'new life' as too painful or dramatic. On the other hand, too slow a rate of change and the client may feel that nothing is happening. Most of us resist change. It needs, perhaps, to be introduced slowly, reinforced often and, most of all, practised. This process is not dissimilar to learning to play an instrument. The more we practise working at change, the better we are likely to be at it. Nor is the change that emerges out of a counselling relationship a once-and-for-all thing. It is likely that most of us very frequently have to review our lives and make adjustments and alterations or, perhaps, learn to acknowledge that certain things about us and our lives cannot be changed. In this case, we need to be able to learn acceptance.

WHO SHOULD COUNSEL?

As we have noted, in a sense, everyone is involved in counselling at some level. On the other hand, not everyone would formally call themselves 'counsellors'. In an effort to answer the question 'Who should be trained as counsellors?', Pearce (1989) offers this useful list for consideration.

- Counselling skills training should be a normal and necessary part of the training of all professionals. The depth of training in those skills is likely to be greater for those engaged in the helping professions such as nursing, teaching and social work than those who are lawyers, dentists, estate agents and so on. An appendix of this book offers the British Association for Counselling's guidelines for the training and registration of counsellors.
- At a lower level, the foundation for counselling skills training should be laid in schools with an increasing emphasis on providing training for students in active listening and on helping them to understand and practise the concepts of respect, empathy and genuineness which contribute towards building effective relationships.
- Managers in industry and elsewhere need counselling skills training in order to understand how counselling integrates with their other functions in working with people.

Elsewhere, counselling has been advocated in at least the following settings.

- Helping those with serious disabilities (Herbert, 1996; Mullins *et al.*, 1997).

- Sex education for young people (O'Driscoll, 1997).
- Empowering oncology rehabilitation patients (Smith *et al.*, 1998).
- Enabling student midwives (Crowley, 1997).
- Preparing people for retirement (Langer, 1997).
- Enabling older people to cope with change (Sennott-Miller and Kligman, 1992).
- Informing people about contraception (Moskowitz and Jennings, 1996).
- Breaking bad news (Winbolt, 1997).
- Teaching spiritual care to health care students (Gallia, 1996; Ross, 1996; Bradshaw, 1997).
- Health promotion amongst those who are HIV in the community (DiScenza *et al.*, 1996).
- Helping people to cope with bereavement (Youll and Wilson, 1996).
- Identifying those who are HIV positive and who are suicidal (Miller, 1995).
- Helping those who are incontinent (Langley, 1995).
- Advising in dietetics (Licavoli and Hahn, 1995).
- Coping with sudden infant death syndrome (McClain and Mandell, 1994).
- Helping with giving up smoking (Hurt *et al.*, 1994; Leininger and Earp, 1993).
- Helping to educate those working in the cancer and palliative care fields (Faulkner *et al.*, 1991).

THE ETHICAL DIMENSION

All health professionals work in situations in which others have to trust them. Those who counsel or use counselling skills are also in positions of considerable trust. Often they will be listening to people who are very vulnerable or listening to stories which are very personal. It is essential that anyone who undertakes counselling or uses counselling skills does so ethically and does not abuse their situation in any way. The British Association for Counselling lays down ethical guidelines for counsellors and for those using counselling skills and these are reproduced as an appendix to this book. It is notable, too, that almost all health professions have their own codes of conduct which will apply just as much to the use of counselling skills as to any other aspects of care or work with clients.

One aspect of maintaining an ethical relationship involves the ability of those using counselling skills to monitor themselves. Counselling relationships often become close. It always remains the responsibility of the health professional using counselling skills to ensure that a reasonable and therapeutic distance is maintained. Without that distance, boundaries – both professional and personal – can become blurred. It is often when this blurring of boundaries occurs that ethical dilemmas arise. This is not to suggest that health professionals and clients should not become close but simply to acknowledge that there is an important difference between a personal relationship and a professional one. In a personal relationship, usually, two people meet as equals in status and they choose, jointly, whether or not to enter into a deeper relationship with each other. This is not the case in a professional relationship, where one person is already designated 'a professional' and, by definition, is expected by the other person to be professional, reliable and trustworthy.

The literature on counselling and therapy contains reports of counsellors and clients who fall in love with one another. It is possible to argue, though, that such relationships are never equality but are based rather more on a power dynamic, with the counsellor always being in a 'one-up' position in relation to the client. It is also possible to argue that the client falls in love with the counsellor as counsellor and not as just another human being. Later in such a relationship, both would have to realize that the original designations of 'client' and 'counsellor' are no longer there and that each is, arguably, not in love with the person they perceived the other to be when they occupied those roles. From being in a 'one-up, one-down' power relationship, they suddenly have to face each other as equals and, arguably, the 'healing' aspect of the relationship is potentially lost as the counsellor becomes just another person with many of their own personal and life problems.

Nor is it simply a case of dismissing the power relationship and declaring that 'I treat my clients as equals, anyway'. This may or may not be the case but it does not allow for how each client may perceive the counsellor or health professional. Simply by being a helper or carer, the health professional is already cast in a certain light by the client. This is not to suggest, in any way, that counsellors and health professionals have 'special powers' in any sense but to acknowledge that they are always acting out a role that is constantly being defined for them by their clients and by themselves.

COUNSELLING AND THE HEALTH PROFESSIONAL

Counselling involves listening, helping, empowering and befriending. In these respects, it is the central feature of the work of all health professionals. Examples of the application of counselling skills are numerous and some are identified below, although the lists are not exhaustive.

1 Medicine

- Helping patients and clients to describe their symptoms.
- Helping clients experiencing emotional, social and relationship problems.
- Facing family crises and difficulties.
- Helping and empowering the 'worried well'.
- Advising people who are worried about HIV/AIDS.

2 *Nursing*

- Helping to plan nursing care.
- Identifying patients' needs and wants.
- Coping with dying and bereaved people.
- Reassuring relatives and colleagues.
- Handling other people's anger and fear.
- Helping students to work through Project 2000 courses.

3 *Occupational therapy*

- Talking through personal issues with clients, individually and in groups.
- Discussing coping strategies.
- Enabling clients to regain their ability to live independently.
- Helping clients to talk about their reactions to their disabilities.

4 *Physiotherapy*

- Helping clients to adapt to long-term disability.
- Helping people to cope with their treatment.
- Helping people to regain their motivation in the rehabilitation process.

5 *Teaching*

- Talking through course work and academic problems.
- Helping students to write essays and dissertations.
- Vocational guidance.
- Pastoral work.

6 *Voluntary work*

- Listening to clients' problems in living.
- Supporting other health professionals.
- Coping with other people's emotional release.
- Learning more about yourself.

7 *Social work*

- Enabling the client and family group to clarify problems and identify goals.
- Helping parents and their children.
- Enabling client advocacy.

8 Speech therapy

- Discussing problems with clients.
- Talking to parents and other relatives.
- Working with other health professionals.

Many of these aspects of health professionals' roles overlap with each other and interrelate between professions. It is also clear, though, that counselling skills form an integral part of the daily work of all health professionals. The skills described and discussed in this book will enable all professionals to enhance their daily practice, whatever their particular focus. Thus the skills may be used by nurses working with the elderly and the mentally ill as well as by those working in rehabilitation and general medicine. Physiotherapists will find the sections on listening, client-centred counselling and coping with emotion useful when helping both the acutely and chronically ill. Occupational therapists may find that what are described as counselling skills in this book are skills that can be used daily when working with both the individual and the group in psychiatric and general practice.

Davis and Fallowfield (1991) identified the following list of 'deficiencies in professional communication' which they use to preface their work on developing counselling skills in the health professions. They offer a useful set of points to consider in the context of any health care professional's work.

1. Failure to greet the patient appropriately, to introduce themselves and to explain their own actions.
2. Failure to elicit easily available information, especially major worries and expectations.
3. Acceptance of imprecise information and the failure to seek clarification.
4. Failure to check the doctor's understanding of the situation against the patient's.
5. Failure to encourage questions or to answer them appropriately.
6. Neglect of covert and overt cues provided verbally or otherwise by the patient.
7. Avoidance of information about the persona, family and social situation, including problems in these areas.
8. Failure to elicit information about the patient's feelings and perceptions of the illness.
9. Directive style with closed questions predominating, frequent interruptions and failure to let the patient talk spontaneously.
10. Focusing too quickly without hypothesis testing.
11. Failure to provide information adequately about diagnosis, treatment, side-effects or prognosis or to check subsequent understanding.
12. Failure to understand from the patient's point of view and hence to be supportive.

13 Poor reassurance.

Although their list refers to 'doctors' and 'patients', Davis and Fallowfield's points could be applied to any health care situation and any set of relationships between health care professionals and the people with whom they work.

VARIETIES OF COUNSELLING

In order to identify the various of aspects of the counselling process, it is useful to identify different sorts of counselling. Counselling is not one set of skills to be used in a narrow range of situations but a differing and often idiosyncratic mixture of personal qualities, practical skills and interpersonal verbal and non-verbal behaviours that combine to make up a particularly caring aspect of the health professional's job. Later, it will be necessary to consider the counsellor's need to take care of themselves: human caring of the sort being described here takes its toll. We cannot be involved with others without that contact touching our own lives, our belief and value systems and our emotional make-up. Counselling is a remarkably personal activity which changes not only the client but also the counsellor. As carers, we need to take care of ourselves.

Supportive counselling

One of the most common forms of counselling is when we are asked to support people. This may take the form of acting as a sounding board for their ideas, plans or suggestions. The primary skill required in acting in this way is that of listening. To really listen to another person is the most caring action of all. Listening is more fully discussed in Chapter 6, in which various aspects of the listening process are explored and the reader is offered practical suggestions on how to improve their listening skills. Whilst we all have experience in listening, so we all have experience of only half listening – of being caught up with our own concerns and of rehearsing our answers. All these things distract us from the process of offering true support to another person. If we are to offer supportive counselling, we must learn to give ourselves almost completely to the other person for the period we are with them – Not really an easy task.

Supportive counselling also calls for more than just the ability to listen. It calls for the capacity to imagine how the world seems to the other person. It is to offer what Rogers (1983) called 'empathic understanding'. This is similar to the old Indian idea that you shouldn't criticize a person without having first walked a mile in his moccasins. To support is also to understand what the other person is feeling. The degree to which it is possible to offer this sort of empathy is open to question and this, too, is taken up in a later chapter.

Another important aspect of any discussion about offering support on a professional basis is the question of *commitment* to the process. Alistair Campbell discusses this issue eloquently, in his book *Paid to Care*

(Campbell, 1984). There seems to be something curious about the fact that we are involved in caring for others in a way that involves deep understanding, whilst also doing a job of work. As users of counselling skills, we need to consider our motives. Whilst altruism and true caring for the needs of others must be part of the counselling process, it is reasonable to assume that in supporting others, we are also getting something out of the process for ourselves. Social exchange theory offers the slightly cynical view that there is always a 'pay-off' in human relationships. Homans (1961) goes as far as to suggest that:

> ***The open secret of human exchange is to give to the other man behaviour that is more valuable to him than it is costly to you and to get from him behaviour that is more valuable to you than it is costly to him.***

Nothing, perhaps, is free. We need to be clear about our motives when offering support and clear about why we are offering support to the other person. If it is part of a professional commitment and part of our job, then we need to work through the implications of that, too. We need to make sure that we can be both sincere in our work and fully aware of the cost as well as the benefits to ourselves.

Supportive counselling occurs in a variety of settings. The physiotherapist who sees a client through the lengthy rehabilitation process is also offering a type of supportive counselling. It is she who often has to listen to the client's darker thoughts and feelings, during the inevitable troughs in the process of rehabilitation. The voluntary worker in a general hospital often undertakes supportive counselling as a very specific part of her role. Very often, she has the time that other health care professionals do not have (or claim not to have). Also, perhaps, because she is doing the job 'for love', her motives for supporting may be clearer. She is taking on the role of counsellor simply because she wants to. General practitioners, in allowing their patients to verbalize their personal and family problems, are also offering supportive counselling. Student nurses in a wide range of settings, from working with the mentally handicapped to caring for the terminally ill, regularly face situations in which they are asked to be supportive.

All health professionals have to help patients and clients adapt to various situations, from learning to live with paralysis to coping with a colostomy. In many of these situations, patients and clients have to adjust to a different body image, a changed perception of self. Fortunately, such adaptation can be made but the health professional who is able to offer adequate and appropriate support can do much to smooth the process.

The skills outlined in this book can enable health professionals to survive the pressures of such situations. Health care, particularly in the UK, has changed dramatically in the past ten years. The provision of care, the means of financing it, the numbers of people involved as carers – all these factors have put pressure on health care professionals as well as on the clients who are recipients of care. Such factors can be emotionally exhausting and undermining. In the past, it was usual to encourage health professionals to 'grin and bear it', to hide their feelings whenever possible. Today, the situation is somewhat paradoxical. On the one hand, there is intense pressure on health professionals to economize and make sure that they offer 'value for money'. On the other, they are more readily encouraged to express their feelings about caring. Thus the 'hardnosed' and the 'softer' approaches seem to have come together. We all have to be sound business people and, at the same time, remember our humanity and frailty.

Informative counselling

Health professionals develop a considerable amount of knowledge about the domain in which they work. Some of this is 'formal' knowledge: knowledge learned from books, lectures and through the educational processes of colleges and universities. Lots of it, though, is 'experiential' or personal knowledge gained through the process of living and working with other people. Much of this knowledge relates directly to how people function and feel. Different sorts of health practitioners have different sorts of very specific knowledge about physiology, disease and health. Many have a wealth of 'ingrained' knowledge that involves intuition as well as rationality. Clients often ask for very specific information about the nature of their health or lack of it and such information is what makes up informative counselling. Clearly, the client requires accurate and understandable information and information on which he can act. A current example of how people may require informative counselling is in the field of HIV and AIDS. People need an understanding of how they should conduct their sexual relationships or manage the administration of intravenous drugs. All of this requires a considerable knowledge base. It is not a simple matter of knowing about using condoms or needle exchange schemes; it is just as much about relationships, both gay and straight, and about people's feelings and fears.

People then, need information. Someone else has that information. All that is left is for the information to be handed over. In reality, of course, it is rarely as simple as that. Any information concerning me and my body or my life concerns me, not in a detached, academic way but in a very personal sense. Anyone who has been a patient in hospital or who has been given advice in a GP's surgery will know the difference between what information 'means' to the medical profession and what it means to the person who is hearing it. Thus, the giving of information, in the health professions, is unlike the giving of information in, say, estate agency. In the latter, we are dealing, at least to some degree, with impersonal, objective facts. In the former situation, the case is overloaded with an emotional aspect that calls at once for sympathy, empathy, tact and considerable skill. To give another person information about themselves or their relatives is an emotional process. Whilst the information must be accurate, the delivery of that information must be appropriate to the needs of the receiver.

Another problem arises here. Giving information about illness, health or physiology seems to be reasonably straightforward if we develop the skill of giving it sensitively. With problems in living, alluded to above, the situation is different. When it comes to giving another person information about how to live their life, we are on much less certain ground. Some would argue that the only person who is truly able to furnish information about someone's problems in living is the person themselves. It would seem prudent to avoid offering information about other people's life situations unless it is directly asked for by the client and then only tentatively. The temptation is often great to suggest to clients what *we* think they should do. Or perhaps we offer them suggestions as to what we would do given their situation. Such advice is not usually very helpful but, fortunately, rarely dangerous. People are relatively self-protecting in this respect and they do not accept advice that they cannot use. On the other hand, this may be a reflection of the way in which clients choose their counsellor. Jean-Paul Sartre (1973) suggested that one person goes to another for advice already knowing the sort of advice that they will receive. They may not do this consciously, but this process of selection does take place on some deeper level. As a demonstration of this, in your own life, reflect on whom you would choose to talk to about the following: problems about money; sexual problems; problems of self-confidence. Now ask yourself what sort of advice you would expect to receive from the people you have chosen. It seems likely that you select the people who will tell you what (at some level or another) you already know.

Informative counselling, then, is best restricted to relatively concrete situations, where expert information can make a direct contribution to the person's well-being. This is rarely the case: better and more effective methods of counselling exist and the skills involved in these methods are easily learned. However, there are exceptions to all this and these are also explored in a later chapter.

It should be noted, too, that just because someone is given up-to-date and expert advice does not automatically mean that the person will take and act on that advice. Being given information does not, necessarily, lead to behaviour change. A good example of this is in the field of smoking. Although most people, today, are offered detailed accounts of why smoking is bad for you, those accounts do not, of themselves, automatically lead to the giving up of smoking. There are plenty of examples of health care professionals who know all the reasons not to smoke and yet continue to do so. There is even a possibility that people experience 'information overload' in the health care services. Most drugs carry lengthy descriptions of what those drugs contain, how they should be used and how they should not be used. Pharmacists, who dispense those drugs, give out further information when the drugs are purchased. It seems possible that a person may find themselves overloaded and even confused by being given so much information and in such a short space of time. Similarly, many doctors have now been trained to 'explain' everything that is to happen to a patient. There remains little evidence, to date, that such information giving either relieves anxiety or leads to behavioural change, even though the motives behind such information giving are benign.

Informative counselling in practice

Sally is a physiotherapist who is visiting an elderly patient, Jean Andrews, in the ward prior to her having a hip replacement operation. During the process of being taught breathing exercises, Jean asks Sally about her operation. Sally uses client-centred counselling interventions to establish what Jean has and has not been told about her coming operation. She is then able to offer clear and precise information about what may be expected, being careful not to use jargon nor to 'talk down' to Jean. In this way, Jean's anxieties are relieved and she is better prepared for her operation because of her increased knowledge. There is evidence to suggest that patients who are given sufficient information about surgery and its possible outcomes suffer subjectively less pain than do those who are not prepared in this way (Hayward, 1975). In this example, too, the information given is of a concrete and practical nature that will enhance the patient's comfort and relieve her anxiety.

Educational counselling

Health professionals are often to be found in educational settings. Most of the professions employ people trained in those professions as educators to the next generation. A number of the caring professions operate an apprenticeship type of training in which work in the field is combined with blocks of academic study. This format, however, is changing rapidly. The nursing profession, for example, used to use an apprenticeship approach to training but has replaced it with a scheme in which all trainee nurses are full-time students in colleges and universities and spend short periods in clinical practice with supernumerary status.

People who work in an educational capacity frequently find themselves in the role of personal tutor to one or more students. Such tutoring combines both the educational aspect of the student's life and the personal. It is this dual function that can combine both types of counselling discussed above – the supportive and the informative. It is usually useful, however, to establish some parameters to the student–tutor relationship and the use of a *contract* is helpful here.

In contract setting, the tutor negotiates the following with the student.

- The amount of time that they will spend together (e.g. one hour per week).
- The type of counselling relationship that is required (e.g. academic and course related and/or personal).
- Whether or not some of the academic counselling will take place in small groups to include other personal tutees. Whilst this may not suit all students, it is certainly more economical in terms of the tutor's time.
- What both student and tutor expect of the relationship.

There are occasions on which the personal aspects of a student's life will shade into their academic life. On the other hand, keeping a counselling conversation focused on one or other of these topics can enable both tutor and student to clarify what they want from the relationship at that particular time. Hopefully, too, the distinction can enable some objectivity about a student's academic work to be maintained by the tutor, although this can be a problem. When personal issues are discussed alongside academic issues, assessing written and project work can become difficult as the tutor may be too distracted by the personal issues involved. In some cases, this may constitute an argument for personal tutors being concerned with academic and work-related issues only. Some might argue that if such tutors begin to help on personal issues, then they are likely to lose the ability to be objective about the student's academic work. To this end, many colleges and universities employ student counsellors who help students with personal issues. Unfortunately, it remains the case that such counsellors are sometimes stigmatized: some students still see it as something of a personal weakness if they have to consult the college counsellor. The ideal picture, perhaps, is of a personal tutor who can move freely between academic, work and personal issues, whilst retaining a certain objectivity about course work. This is, in practice, harder than it sounds.

The skills of educational counselling and coaching are very similar to those of other sorts of counselling. This was illustrated, quite dramatically, by the late psychologist George Kelly, in his description of the various facets of his work as a teacher and therapist.

> ***One of my tasks in the 1930s was to direct graduate studies leading to the Master's Degree. A typical afternoon might find me talking to a graduate student at one o'clock, doing all those familiar things that thesis directors have to do – encouraging the student to pin-point the issues, to observe, to become intimate with the problem, to form hypotheses either inductively or deductively, to control his experiments so that he will know what led to what, to generalise cautiously and to revise his thinking in the light of experience.***
>
> ***At two o'clock I might have an appointment with a client. During this interview I would not be taking the role of the scientist but rather helping the distressed person work out some solutions to his life's problems. So what would I do? Why, I would try to get him to pin-point the issues, to observe, to become intimate with the problem, to form hypotheses, to make test runs, to relate outcomes to anticipations, to control his ventures so that he will know what led to what, to generalise cautiously and to revise his dogma in the light of experience . . . (Kelly, 1963)***

So was born Kelly's personal construct theory, in which Kelly maintained that 'people are scientists' who are continuously developing hypotheses about how they and the world around them will be and then testing those hypotheses against how the world actually turns out.

Counselling in crisis

Another aspect of counselling is helping the person who suddenly finds himself in crisis. Murgatroyd and Woolfe (1982) have characterized a crisis in the following ways.

- Symptoms of stress – the person experiences stress both physically and psychologically.
- Attitude of panic or defeat – the person feels overcome by the situation and experiences both helplessness and hopelessness.
- Focus on relief – the person wants, more than anything else, relief from the feeling of being in crisis.
- Lowered efficiency – in other areas of their life, apart from the crisis, the person's functioning may be impaired.
- Limited duration – because the experience is psychologically painful, it does not last long and can be viewed as an acute experience of limited duration.

There are many different sorts of crises that occur in people's lives, ranging from sudden death to the realization of child abuse in a family. Differences occur, too, with regard to the point at which individuals perceive themselves to be in crisis. Thus, the point at which counselling interventions are offered will vary from person to person. Sometimes that intervention is offered through access to a crisis intervention team of one sort or another. Usually such teams are multidisciplinary and offer the services of a range of practitioners. At other times, crisis counselling is offered through telephone counselling and through a range of helplines. Clearly, telephone counselling calls for a very different range of skills from face-to-face counselling, in that all non-verbal means of communication between the two people are lost and verbal intervention is almost the only means of interchange available. The word 'almost' is used deliberately here, for even on the telephone, an intuitive sense of a situation may be grasped by the effective counsellor. General guidelines in counselling on the telephone include the following.

- Allow the caller to talk freely. Try not to interrupt them but keep them talking.
- Take the lead from the caller. Explore the issues they want to talk about.
- Once you have established rapport, try to make sure that the caller (or other people in their company) are out of direct danger.
- Use occasional 'minimal prompts' to indicate that you are listening ('mm' or 'yes') but use them sparingly.
- If appropriate, make sure that you have the caller's name and a contact phone number. Make sure that the caller knows your name.

Crisis counselling calls for swift action in helping the person to function effectively. Schwartz (cited by Murgatroyd, 1986) offers some suggestions as to how such action may be initiated. Amongst other things, Schwartz suggests the following steps that the counsellor may take.

- Help the person face up to the crisis – discourage denial and try to help them to be objective.
- Break up the crisis into manageable doses – most people can deal with serious problems more easily if they are not overwhelmed by the sheer magnitude of the situation.
- Avoid false reassurance – the counsellor should resist the temptation to prematurely assure the person in crisis that 'everything will work out OK'.
- Help and encourage the person to help themselves – if the person in crisis can actively use the help of friends or family this will cut down the dependence on the counsellor and increase decision making.
- Teach the person in crisis coping skills – once the immediate danger has past, the individual needs to develop a repertoire of coping strategies to help ward off future similar situations.

Crisis counselling is demanding work and the urgency of the situation often calls for quick decisions to be made. In such situations, it is easy for the counsellor to try to take control of the situation. Whilst this may help in the first instance, such an approach does not help the person in crisis in the longer term. Sometimes, crisis counselling calls for considerable constraint on the part of the counsellor and it is often emotionally draining. For this reason, it is often helpful, wherever possible, for crisis counselling to be conducted in pairs or by a small group of people. In this way, mutual support is offered by the counsellors to each other, the responsibility for the situation is shared and more objective help can be offered. However crisis counselling is organized, the counsellor should have available a list of names and telephone numbers of other agencies who may be able to help. Knowing that you have a referral number to the local social services, police, rape crisis centre or other agency means that you are more readily able to offer concrete and practical help to defuse the situation.

There are numerous examples of crises that health care professionals may have to help their clients or patients through and a short list of such crises would include, at least, the following:

- rape or sexual assault;
- sudden death of a partner or spouse;
- child abuse;
- sudden death of a child;
- trauma caused by accident or injury;
- sudden onset of acute psychological or emotional distress;
- suicide or attempted suicide;
- fear of death or the process of dying;

- concern about HIV/AIDS;
- fear of surgical intervention;
- sudden and acute physical pain;
- acute anxiety about the future;
- panic attacks.

Post-trauma counselling

In the past few years, as in other decades and centuries, we have witnessed large-scale wars, disasters and personal tragedies. The sort of counselling that is undertaken to help someone after a major trauma is similar, in a way, to that used to help the bereaved (Parkinson, 1993). Parkinson suggests that there are four main tasks in post-trauma counselling.

1. To help people to accept the reality of their experiences and to counteract the defence of denial.
2. To encourage them to feel the pain and to provide reassurance of the normality of their reactions. This also deals with the problem of denial.
3. To help them adjust and adapt to the changes which have taken place in their lives.
4. To help them redirect their emotions and their lives so that they can move to acceptance and healing.

In the end, as in all forms of counselling, the person has to find their own way through. Brian Keenan, a hostage in the Middle East for nearly five years, wrote the following in an article in *The Guardian* on Friday August 9th 1991, soon after the release of his friend and fellow hostage, John McCarthy.

> ***Each man must find within himself the various methods to contain and control the pain and confusion within. There are no ready-made answers. It is a slow process of rediscovery, where denial or flight from the inward turmoil is the antithesis of self-healing. We go that road alone. We may be helped but we cannot be pushed or misdirected. We each have the power within us to re-humanise ourselves. We are our own self-healers.***

Keenan was writing about the after effects of trauma but he might have been writing about anyone who experiences profound personal and emotional problems and his words summarize well the central issue in counselling: self-healing.

There is a question here, too, about time. It is possible to believe, from the media, that people require counselling *immediately* after a tragedy. It is arguable, however, that people, in some situations, may need time in order to reflect on what has happened to them and to allow the healing processes of rationalization to take their course. Perhaps people do not always need immediate counselling after a life-shattering event.

Counselling in spiritual distress

Spiritual distress is the result of a total inability to invest life with meaning. It can be demotivating and painful and can cause anguish to the sufferer. Counselling people who experience such distress presents a considerable challenge to health professionals who care for them.

It would seem that the need to find meaning in what we do is a very basic human need (Bugental and Bugental, 1984). Such meaning may be framed in the context of religious beliefs that can take very varied forms (Wallis, 1984). Alternatively, meaning may be found through adherence to a particular ideological viewpoint: philosophical, psychological, sociological or political. Others take the view expressed by Kopp (1974) that there is no meaning to life except what we as individuals invest in it. Those with a positivistic scientific view of the world may dismiss the metaphysical altogether and thus the notion of a spiritual problem does not arise for them. We should, of course, be open to this too. Not everyone needs spiritual care nor finds the world of the spiritual of importance to them.

The first qualification for engaging in spiritual counselling may be the development of an understanding of a wide range of religious doctrines, philosophical and political systems of thought and an appreciation of how various thinkers throughout history have approached the ultimate questions of life. Such an enterprise can be humbling. It can enable us to understand that not everyone views the world as we do and may guard against any temptation on the part of the counsellor to proselytize. As Jung pointed out (Fordham, 1966), the counsellor needs to be a 'wise' person, not only trained in counselling methods but also widely read, experienced and open-minded.

Counsellors also need a highly developed intuitive sense: the ability to see and understand beyond the words that people use to attempt to express themselves. Carl Rogers (1967) noted that he felt himself to be functioning best as a counsellor when he paid full attention to this intuitive sense.

Counselling in the spiritual domain, then, is far more than the development of a range of counselling skills. It involves the whole person and can, at times, tax the counsellor's own beliefs and value system. Indeed, the counsellor must be prepared to 'live on the edge' when counselling in spiritual distress and acknowledge that there are times when there are no answers to the taxing problems of meaning.

Who, then, are the people likely to require spiritual counselling? The range of those who experience spiritual problems is wide and includes adolescents suffering from identity crises (Erikson, 1959) to those in middle age who may suddenly be faced with the difficulty of individuation (Storr, 1983) to the older person who may fear death. Along this age dimension are those of any age who suddenly find themselves confronting the issue of personal meaning. This may happen as part of a depressive illness but it may also happen when depression is not present. Dispiritedness or the failure to find meaning has been described as a state of mind separate from depression and identified as the questioning of the point of life in someone who is otherwise functioning 'normally' (Tillich, 1952; Bugental, 1980). It may occur, for instance, in the person who up to that point has held well-defined religious beliefs but who now has doubts about them. It can happen in those who are faced with some extreme challenge in life and are left questioning the reasons for such an occurrence. It can occur, also, as a result of the crisis described in the previous section and should be looked for as a possibility after the immediate crisis has abated. Clearly, it can occur in a great number of situations that are found in hospitals: during sudden, severe and life-threatening illness; following surgical intervention that causes changes in body image (mastectomy, for example); following the death of a child or a close relative; and numerous other situations in which the person may call into question the issue of meaning.

In later life, the problem of individuation, described by Jung (Storr, 1983) as the quest for finding and understanding the self, may be preceded by a feeling of vacuum, pointlessness and lack of self-motivation. The psychoanalyst Victor Frankl has described this feeling as an 'existential vacuum' (Frankl, 1959, 1969, 1975). He argues that this is characterized by despair, distress and a feeling of emptiness. Frankl is clear, however, that this is not a neurotic condition but a very common human experience. Indeed, such a feeling is well described in works of literature that are concerned with the human condition. It occurs in the hero of Sartre's *Nausea* (1965) and Hesse's *Steppenwolf* (1927) and is addressed extensively in Colin Wilson's survey of such literature, *The Outsider* (Wilson, 1955). It is the darker side of the human situation.

The whole issue of dispiritedness, existential vacuum or spiritual collapse presents a great challenge to the health professional who meets people suffering from such life crises. How, then, may we help the person who, almost by definition, seems beyond counselling? Perhaps the first thing that we can do is to *listen* to the person. When we are threatened by the content of another person's conversation, it is tempting to refuse to let them talk. Somehow, the despairing content of their conversation seems to call into question our own beliefs about life.

This may indeed be the case and it suggests that before we engage in counselling of any sort, we therefore clarify our own belief and value systems (Simon *et al.*, 1978). If we are clearer about our own view of life, we may find that we are less threatened by the views of others. There is, however, no guarantee. We enter into every spiritual counselling situation as something of an act of faith; there can be no absolute certainty that we will not be changed by the encounter. It may be important that this is so. If we are so secure in our own belief system, we may also become closed minded and less questioning: such a position is probably not the best one from which to work as a counsellor.

Apart from listening to the person who is experiencing spiritual distress, we need also to *accept* what they say. If someone expresses particularly negative thoughts, the temptation is to try to persuade them to think otherwise. In counselling, however, the aim is to listen and to accept and not to argue. Often this means that the person being counselled needs to quietly talk through something, sit in silence for some time and generally to acknowledge and face the blankness that they feel. Often, the very facing of the blankness can lead to an apparent paradoxical change. It is as though through allowing and accepting the feeling, the feeling itself changes. Sometimes those who face complete meaninglessness find meaning. This accent on accepting rather than fighting feelings is described in detail by Reibel (1984) who calls it the homeopathic approach to counselling. She adopts the metaphor of homeopathy to describe this process of 'allowing' a condition or state of mind rather than fighting it. In homeopathic medicine, minute doses of toxins that cause an illness are given as a remedy for that illness. So, in homeopathic counselling, the thoughts and feelings that are troubling the spiritually distressed person are encouraged rather than argued against. Sometimes, by such encouragement the dispirited feelings are transformed or transmuted and replaced by more positive, life-asserting feelings.

Closely allied to this homeopathic approach is that which involves the use of paradoxical strategies. These are variously described as paradoxical intention (Frankl, 1960, 1975), paradoxical interventions (Tennen *et al.*, 1981) and paradoxical therapy (Fay, 1978, 1986). These constitute a cluster of techniques whose essential element is an unexpected reversal of the anticipated procedure. Thus, instead of joining forces with the client to tackle his dispiritedness, the practitioner suggests a continuance or even an intensification of the negative feelings. This curious about-turn in counselling can, again, sometimes encourage a contrary alleviation of the negative feelings. It is as though on being implored to get worse, the client gets better! On the other hand, such an approach will not work with everyone, nor will it suit every practitioner.

This is perhaps the crux of spiritual counselling and, for that matter, of any sort of counselling – that no one approach works for everyone. Health professionals engaged in spiritual counselling need to remain sensitive to personal needs and differences. Indeed, if they can develop the deeper listening approach alluded to previously and described in more detail in Chapter 5, they may enter the client's world view and discover, through the client, the right approach. The client, in other words, is telling the counsellor what help they need. The difficulty lies in being receptive to that description. There are times when clients have great difficulty in articulating what their needs are, but such articulation is nearly always possible given time and sensitivity and also a considerable amount of humility on the part of the counsellor.

Health professionals acting as counsellors always need to know their limitations. They need to know when to call in other help agents, whether those agents are doctors, clergy, other members of the family or other health professionals. There are times, too, when counsellors have too close a relationship with the client and find their own judgement clouded by this closeness. If they are supported by other colleagues, such a period can be worked through to the benefit of both client and counsellor.

The skills involved in counselling the person who is spiritually distressed may serve as a template for the sorts of skills required in all counselling situations. Perhaps because of the extreme nature of the person's feelings, counselling in this situation calls upon certain aspects that we shall encounter again and again in later chapters: the ability to listen, to accept and to have some self-understanding.

It should be noted, too, that the word 'spiritual', used in this context, is not necessarily synonymous with the word 'religious'. Spiritual concerns, as they are described here, are concerns about *meaning*. the quest for meaning is probably a universal one and is just as much the domain of agnostics and atheists as it is of believers. On the other hand, McLeod (1998) notes counselling's historical links with religion, as follows.

> ***Another field of study which has a strong influence on counselling theory and practice is religion. Several counselling agencies have begun their life as branches of the Church, or have been helped into existence by founders with a religious calling. Many of the key figures in the history of counselling and psychotherapy have had strong religious backgrounds, and have attempted to integrate the work of the counsellor with the search for spiritual meaning. Jung made the most significant contribution in this area. Although the field of counselling is permeated with Judaeo-Christian thought and belief, there is increasing interest among some counselling in the relevance of ideas and practices from other religions, such as Zen Buddhism.***

Counselling in spiritual distress in practice

Siân is a senior nurse in a large psychiatric hospital. Whilst talking to Ann, a ward sister, during her staff appraisal meeting, she discovers that Ann finds it difficult to sustain interest in her work as the head of an acute admissions ward. At first, this lack of motivation appears to be a result of having worked on the ward for two years. After further discussion, however, Ann talks of her difficulty in seeing the 'point' of her work and talks of a general disenchantment with life itself. Siân and Ann meet regularly and Ann is allowed to talk through her feelings. Gradually, she discovers a sense of purpose again, although there are times when both Siân and Ann are uncertain about the possible outcome of their discussions. Siân notes, too, that earlier in her career as a psychiatric nurse, she would have tended to dismiss Ann's problem as a symptom of depression.

Counselling in emotional distress

Frequently, there are times when the counselling relationship evokes emotion in the client. Sometimes this arises out of the discussion that the client is having; the very nature of the material under discussion is painful and brings to the surface many bottled-up feelings. At other times, the client comes to the practitioner in distress.

In the first instance, when the client is stirred up by the nature of the discussion, the most helpful thing that the counsellor can do is to allow the full expression of those feelings (Heron, 1977a). As we have seen in the previous section, this allowing goes against the cultural grain. We are more readily moved to cheer the person up or to help them to stop expressing strong feeling, even more so when that person's expression of emotion stirs up feelings in us. It is arguable, however, that it is exactly because the person has been encouraged to bottle things up that they perceive themselves as having problems. It is as though the bottled-up emotion tends to make for more negative perceptions. On the other hand, if those emotions are fully released, the person's perception of the situation will often become more positive. Clearly, this is not always the case. People in all walks of life experience real and distressing situations that cannot easily be resolved: death in the family, unemployment, illness, financial problems and so forth. None of these situations can be changed easily by the process of counselling. Even though this is true, the individual's *perception* of their situation can still change through counselling and, in this case, through expression of pent-up emotion. In a sense, there are no good or bad life situations: what is good and bad is the way in which we view those situations, the sense we make of them. Whilst counselling may not be able to change the fact that much of life is intractable, it can help in encouraging a more positive and life-assertive world view.

When the client comes to the practitioner in a distressed and emotional state, a decision has to be made on whether to distract the person and move them away from their emotional release or whether to accept the release as outlined previously. Much will depend here on what the client is asking of the counsellor. Are they asking for help to control their emotional state? Are they asking that the counsellor hear them and allow them their expression? As we noted in the section on counselling in spiritual distress (p. 19), the counsellor must learn to read the signs and to hear what is being requested. If there is still ambiguity and the client's needs and wants are not clear, the counsellor can ask the client what they want. At first, this may seem like an uncomfortable option. In practice, it is quite possible to say to the other person: 'Do you want to continue crying or would you like me to help you stop?' Again, such an intervention is countercultural. Normally we do not ask such questions! The question can do much to help the client to determine exactly what is needed at this particular time. It is easy to imagine that because a person is crying, they are out of control in every other respect. The person who is crying is still able to be self-determining and make decisions about what it is they do or do not want of another person.

The stranger-on-the-train phenomenon

Perhaps a reason counselling in emotional distress 'works' is that it can feel comfortable disclosing problems to a complete stranger. While it may be difficult to talk to someone you know really well, paradoxically, it can be easy to self-disclose, in some depth, to a complete stranger. Sometimes, the counselling can fulfil the role of the complete stranger. The tendency to disclose in this way has been called the 'stranger-on-the-train' phenomenon and, ironically, it is perhaps best described by the travel writer and novelist, Paul Theroux (1977).

> ***The conversation, like many others I had with people on trains, derived an easy candour from the shared journey, the comfort of the dining car, and the certain knowledge that neither of us would see each other again.***

The specific skills involved in helping the person experiencing emotional release are described in Chapter 7. This section has merely opened up the question of what to do when someone is in emotional distress. Again, it would seem that the accepting method has much to commend it as a style of counselling

Confessional counselling

There are times when people need to talk, in confidence, about things that they feel unable to disclose to anyone else. This might be called confessional counselling and it can take a number of forms. Sometimes, a person has a particular habit or way of thinking that they feel to be somehow 'odd' and they seek reassurance that it is quite OK to be odd. Sometimes, relief comes simply from someone else having 'heard' them – that they have been able to disclose. At other times, the 'confession' may take the form of disclosure of something that proves to contrary to the law – child abuse, certain sexual acts and so on. This type of disclosure may change the dynamics of the counselling relationship for what is said cannot be unsaid. The counsellor, in a very clear way, is to some degree party to the act that has been described. The issue of confidentiality in counselling is discussed later but anyone working in the counselling field should be aware of the possibility of listening to someone who tells them something that places a certain responsibility on them as counsellor. If I tell you that I have committed an obviously illegal act, then you also shoulder some of the responsibility. The act of telling becomes one of sharing responsibility.

The experienced counsellor may well have a strong sense of when such disclosures are being approached. They will need to make a decision about the implications of hearing such a disclosure and may even decide to discuss the implications with the client. It seems reasonable to me to say something to the effect that 'I think you want to tell me something very serious about your life and I want us to talk about the implications of what your telling me might be'.

It must be borne in mind that the counsellor does not stand outside the law and cannot claim immunity for knowing certain things about another person if those things are of an illegal nature. Nor is this a debate about morality in the broader sense. The issue at stake here is whether or not, by knowing something 'illegal' about another person, we are forced to act on that information. An extreme example may help here. If a person were to tell you that they had murdered someone and intended to kill again, you would presumably be in no doubt that action was required to try to prevent this happening. Another example, although perhaps a little less black and white, is the person who discloses that they sometimes have suicidal feelings. In this case, the counsellor must make some sort of judgement about whether or not it is always appropriate to pass this information on to another person. I was once faced, on a Friday evening, with a student who discussed the possibility of suicide. As I was likely to be the last person in the college to see her that afternoon, I had to weigh up what my responsibilities were towards her and towards her family and friends. In the end, I talked her into letting me go with her to her GP.

The point of this debate is to be prepared. The person who counsels or uses counselling skills must have thought through, beforehand, the implications of people telling them things which they may not want to hear.

COUNSELLING CONTEXTS IN THE HEALTH CARE PROFESSIONS

The range of situations in which health care professionals may be called to counsel is vast and no one list is likely to cover every possibility. It is interesting, however, to note the contexts described in Davis and Fallowfield's (1991a) book and to attempt to add to it.

- Counselling and renal failure.
- Counselling and disfigurement.
- Counselling in head injury.
- Counselling with spinal cord-injured people.
- Counselling people with multiple sclerosis and their families.
- Infertility counselling.
- Counselling in gynaecology.
- Genetic counselling.
- Neonatal intensive care counselling.
- Counselling families of children with disabilities.
- Counselling in paediatrics.
- Counselling patients with cancer.
- Counselling in heart disease.

Other contexts that might be added to this list would include, at least, the following.

- HIV and AIDS counselling.
- Counselling gay and bisexual people.
- Counselling in sexual dysfunction.
- Career counselling.
- Racial counselling.
- Counselling in mental health settings.
- Rehabilitation counselling.

COUNSELLING AND PSYCHOTHERAPY

The differences between counselling and psychotherapy are often blurred. Nelson-Jones (1995) offers this distinction.

> ***The term 'counselling' is used in a number of ways. For instance, counselling may be viewed: as a special kind of helping relationship; as a repertoire of interventions; as a psychological process; or in terms of its goals, or the people who counsel, or its relationship to psychotherapy.***

However, Davies (1987) is less sure about the relative differences between the two and she suggests that:

> ***The only difference between definitions of counselling and psychotherapy according to the perspectives of writers such as Nelson-Jones is essentially one of emphasis rather than there being any definitive or absolute differences in the definitions. Differences in emphasis may be seen in the nature of the relations, in the theoretical orientation of the activity, in the setting in which the activity takes place and in the different client populations.***
>
> ***However, even this distinction appears relative rather than absolute. Consider the point about the settings in which counselling and psychotherapy take place: definitions of counselling tend to point out that counselling is more likely to take place in non-medical settings rather than medical settings. In terms of client populations, definitions of counselling tend to indicate that counselling focuses on moderately to severely disturbed clients. However, it should be emphasized that any such distinctions are relative rather than forming mutually exclusive categories. Carl Rogers, himself, worked with clients who had been diagnosed as schizophrenic, while many of the therapies which come under the term psychological therapy, such as the cognitive and behaviour therapies, are viewed frequently as the therapy of choice for less distressed clients. Further, counsellors are increasingly being employed to work in such medical settings as general practice or in health centres, as well as in clinical psychology departments and in psychotherapy departments within the NHS.***
>
> ***Generally, it may still be the case that counsellors in these settings tend to be referred less chronically disturbed clients.***

THE RANGE OF COUNSELLING INTERVENTIONS

Whatever sort of counselling is undertaken, certain skills and processes are involved. Counselling skills can be divided into two groups:

1 listening and attending;
2 verbal counselling interventions.

In other words, the counsellor listens to the client and verbally responds. The skills involved in listening are described more fully in Chapter 6. It may be useful, however, to identify the range of counselling interventions that may be used in any counselling situation. John Heron, a British philosopher and humanistic therapist, has devised a valuable division of all possible therapeutic interventions, called Six-category intervention analysis (Heron, 1986). The analysis transcends any particular theoretical stance adopted by the counsellor and has many applications. The six categories described in Heron's analysis are:

1 prescriptive interventions;
2 informative interventions;
3 confronting interventions;
4 cathartic interventions;
5 catalytic interventions;
6 supportive interventions.

These six categories will be described in further detail but it is important to note that Heron further subdivides the categories into those he calls authoritative (the first three) and those he calls facilitative (the second three). Authoritative counselling interventions are those in which the counsellor plays a directive role in the counselling relationship and guides it in a fairly structured way. Facilitative counselling interventions are those in which the counsellor plays a less directive role and enables the client to take more control over the relationship. Another way of describing the difference is that authoritative interventions are 'I tell you' interventions and facilitative ones are 'you tell me' interventions. Heron argues that the skilled counsellor can use a balance of the two types of interventions appropriately in a wide range of counselling situations. It is not, then, a question of using all the different types of interventions in all counselling situations but of consciously choosing the right intervention for the right occasion. What, then, are examples of the six categories of therapeutic intervention?

Prescriptive interventions

Prescriptive interventions are those in which the counsellor's intention is to suggest or recommend a particular line of action. Thus, if the counsellor says, 'I recommend you talk this over with your family', they are making a prescriptive intervention. Heron suggests that when prescriptive interventions are clumsily used, they can degenerate into heavy-handed, moralistic patronage. Certainly they can easily be overused in counselling.

Examples of how prescriptive interventions may be effective in the health care setting are when a physiotherapist offers a recently paralysed person practical suggestions as to how their mobility may be increased with the use of a wheelchair or offers an elderly person advice about how to use a walking frame correctly.

Informative interventions

Informative interventions are those in which the counsellor informs or instructs the client in some way. If, for example, the health professional says, 'You will probably find that you will have some discomfort in your leg for about three weeks', they are using an informative intervention. Heron notes here that unskilful use of informative interventions leads to dependence on the counsellor and the relationship can degenerate into one of overteaching on the part of the counsellor. As we have seen from the previous discussion on informative counselling, information is best limited to concrete situations and should not extend to 'putting your life right' information.

The nurse who instructs a patient on why they should complete a course of antibiotics is offering informative help. It is notable that such information is limited to concrete, practical issues. As we have seen, it is easy to take over a patient's life and create dependence through offering too much information.

Confronting interventions

Interventions of this sort are those that challenge the client in some way or draw their attention to a particular type of repetitive behaviour. An example of a confronting intervention may be 'I notice that you frequently complain about the way your wife talks to you. . .'. If confrontation is used too frequently in the counselling situation, it may be perceived by the client as an aggressive approach. Clearly, confrontation needs to be used appropriately and sensitively. This issue is addressed more specifically in Chapter 10.

Cathartic interventions

These are interventions that enable the client to release tension through the expression of pent-up emotion. Thus, an intervention that allows a person to cry may be termed cathartic. The counsellor may give the client permission to cry by saying 'You seem to be near to tears . . . it's all right with me if you cry . . .'. Cathartic interventions may be misused when they force the client to release feelings when they are clearly not ready or willing to express them. It is sometimes tempting but rarely appropriate to anticipate that it will 'do the client good' to express bottled-up feeling. More appropriately, perhaps, it should be the client who decides when and if such release of emotion occurs. The issues of emotional release and cathartic skills are discussed in greater detail in Chapter 9.

There are many health care situations in which effective use of cathartic skills is valuable. A short list would include, at least, the following.

- Supporting the recently bereaved person.
- Helping the person who is adjusting to new, and profound disability.
- Assisting people to cope with shock after trauma.

- Helping the person to express their feelings after assault, rape or accident.
- Enabling the depressed person to release pent-up feelings of anger or self-doubt.

All carers need cathartic skills and yet they are perhaps the most difficult to develop. They require considerable self-awareness on the part of the professional and a willingness to explore our own emotional make-up.

Catalytic interventions

Catalytic interventions are those that draw the client out and encourage them to discuss issues further. Thus, any sort of question is an example of a catalytic intervention. Again, used inappropriately, questions can appear interrogative and intrusive; they need to be well timed and sensitively phrased. Certain other forms of catalytic intervention may be more appropriate than questions and these are discussed further in Chapter 7.

Catalytic interventions are perhaps the most useful of all interventions to the health professional. Often it is essential to explore how much a patient or client knows about their condition, prior to offering further information. The person skilled in catalytic counselling can discreetly and tactfully help the person to express their own wants and needs. Thus, catalytic counselling can become an integral part of health care assessment.

Supportive interventions

These are interventions that support, validate or encourage the client in some way. Thus, when the counsellor tells the client, 'I appreciate what you are doing', they are offering a supportive intervention. Used badly, supportive interventions can degenerate into patronage. Often, too, they are symptomatic of the counsellor's need to reassure the client too quickly – perhaps evidence of the counsellor being a 'compulsive helper'.

These, then, are short descriptions of the six categories. Heron (1986) suggests that, as a set of categories, they cover all possible therapeutic interventions. Thus, anything a counsellor can say to a client will fit under one of these six headings.

The category analysis has a number of applications. First, it can help us to appreciate a wide range of possible interventions to use in the counselling relationship. In everyday conversation, we tend to limit ourselves to a particular and often rather limited range of expressions, questions and verbal responses. The category analysis offers the chance to identify other interventions that we could use. Further, we can learn to make use of what Heron (1977b) calls 'conscious use of self'. In other words, we learn to take responsibility for what we say and choose to make a particular intervention at a particular time. At first, this obviously feels unnatural and clumsy. It is, however, the key to becoming an effective and appropriate counsellor. If we do not reflect on what we say and how we say it, we limit our competence. If we consciously choose what we say, then we can broaden our repertoire.

Second, the analysis can make us aware of alternative interventions. There are occasions in counselling, as in every other situation in life, when we may think, 'What do I say now?'. Reference to the category analysis offers further possibilities of response: this must be the case if Heron's claim that it covers all possible therapeutic interventions is valid.

Further, the analysis can be used as a research tool for identifying how groups of people view their own counselling skills. In a study of 93 trained nurses in the UK who were asked to rate themselves on their own perception of their levels of counselling skills using the analysis, most said that they were most effective at being prescriptive, informative and supportive, not as skilled at being catalytic and least skilled at using confronting and cathartic interventions effectively (Burnard and Morrison, 1987). Such research is easily carried out and can be used, at a local level, to determine training needs in the interpersonal domain, in much the same way as has been recommended above.

Becoming aware of the range of counselling skills available is the first step towards becoming an effective counsellor. The next stage is to consider when and how to use those skills effectively.

COUNSELLING OR EVERYDAY COMMUNICATION SKILLS?

In any debate about counselling, the question arises as to when counselling skills can be differentiated from the skills used by a person who is a very effective communicator. Clearly, there is an overlap between the skills of a counsellor and a person with everyday interpersonal skills (see Figure 1.1). The person with 'everyday' skills is likely to be a good listener. They are likely to be able to see the other person's point of view and will be little inclined to force their views on the other person. Perhaps the thing that marks out someone with counselling skills is their ability to focus, almost exclusively, *on the other person*. For this is what counselling involves; it means leaving behind your own interests, opinions, needs and wants and giving your time completely to the other person.

To look at the other side of the argument, it does not follow that the person with counselling skills also has effective interpersonal skills in a range of other settings. It is quite possible to meet people who are useful and helpful to others in the structured, one-to-one atmosphere of the counselling situation but less comfortable dealing with others on a more informal basis or with people in groups. There may be something of a contradiction here. If we argue that the important thing in counselling is an inherent 'humanness' in the counsellor, then we might expect that humanness to spill over into other, everyday situations. Ironically, though, this does not always seem to be the case.

Trying to stand outside the debate for a moment, almost all health care professionals require effective communication and interpersonal skills in order to do their jobs. On the other hand, only relatively few need to be

Acting as an ambassador for the organization
Admitting you were wrong
Answering the phone
Apologizing
Arguing
Attending a tribunal
Avoiding certain topics
Being a go-between
Being an advocate
Breaking bad news
Breaking up arguments
Chairing a conference
Chairing a discussion
Chairing a formal meeting
Chatting
Controlling feelings
Correcting another person
Countering someone else's argument
Criticizing
Defending a colleague
Defending an idea
Defending an opinion
Describing
Disagreeing
Disciplining
Dissuading
Distracting
Encouraging
Expressing feelings
Giving a conference paper
Giving a presentation to colleagues
Giving a report
Giving advice
Giving an opinion
Giving information
Giving instructions
Helping
Instructing
Interrupting
Introducing self
Inviting ideas
Listening
Mediating
Negotiating
Offering a verbal assessment
Participating in a group
Passing judgement
Passing on information
Passing the time of day
Persuading
Reasoning
Receiving bad news
Receiving good news
Rectifying a mistake
Remaining silent
Returning goods
Saying 'no'
Saying 'sorry'
Saying good-bye
Saying good-bye to a group of people
Seeking opinions
Selling an idea
Sharing a joke
Sharing feelings
Sharing good news
Sharing ideas
Sharing self
Sharing thoughts
Showing appropriate anger
Speaking over an intercom system
Sticking to a point of view
Supporting
Supporting relatives
Supporting someone else's argument
Switching your viewpoint
Taking instructions
Talking on radio/television
Talking to patients
Talking to colleagues
Talking to people from other disciplines
Talking to the press
Talking whilst carrying out a procedure
Teaching patients/clients
Teaching peers
Teaching students
Thanking an individual
Thanking people in a group
Using the telephone
Welcoming guests

Figure 1.1

A comprehensive list of interpersonal/communication skills in the health care professions (Burnard, 1996).

skilled as counsellors. In the middle of all this is the value of having both general communication skills and some counselling skills. Presumably, health care professionals who have both these sets of skills are likely to function best of all. I have discussed, in more detail, the acquisition of general interpersonal and communication skills elsewhere (Burnard, 1996, 1997).

THE OUTCOME OF EFFECTIVE COUNSELLING

Clearly, people respond differently to being counselled but it is worth considering what Carl Rogers thought was the general outcome of effective counselling. His list of the changes that may take place is based on observation and evaluation of numerous people 'getting better' in counselling and may serve as a useful indicator of the personal changes that can be achieved.

> ***The person comes to see himself differently. He accepts himself and his feelings more fully. He becomes more self-confident and self-directing. He becomes more flexible, less rigid in his perceptions. He adopts more realistic goals for himself. He behaves in a more mature fashion... He becomes more acceptant of others. He becomes more open to the evidence, both to what is going on outside of himself and to what is going on inside of himself. He changes in his basic personality characteristics in constructive ways. (Rogers, 1967)***

However, we must remember that these were Rogers' observations and not ones based particularly on research. It is possible to view these 'outcomes' as rather too optimistic. In the latter part of the 20th century, it may be reasonable to settle for less. Sometimes, the fact that one part of a person's life has been helped by counselling is enough and sometimes it is all that we can expect. Perhaps, regrettably, there will be times when counselling cannot help and we would do well to bear this in mind too. Counselling can never be a panacea.

2 Psychological approaches to counselling

In the latter part of the 20th century, there is a considerable range of different types of counselling. If we look at advertisements for counsellors, we find that they range from the 'traditional' to the 'new age'. The former will tend to be aligned to particular psychological schools of psychology while the latter will often adopt what they call an 'eclectic' approach, drawing from a range of different perspectives. How 'pure' a psychological approach to counselling should be is a matter of debate, as is the degree to which it is possible to use the word 'eclectic' to mean the equivalent of 'I act as a counsellor in the way that I feel like acting at the time'. Eclecticism could be an excuse for having no particular 'school' to follow or it could be a demonstration of open-mindedness and a willingness to try to offer the client exactly what they need. It is worth taking a little time to reflect on these two possible situations yourself. Which position do you favour: adherence to one particular approach or the use of a number of approaches?

Anyone who acts as a counsellor has certain assumptions about the nature of the person. We all carry with us a certain set of beliefs about the psychological make-up of ourselves and other people. Often, this belief system is only hazily articulated. Sometimes, it is not articulated at all. However vague that system is, it motivates us and helps us in our decision making about how to help other people. In this chapter, some formalized belief systems about the person are briefly explored, drawn from a variety of schools of psychology. It is suggested that in exploring this variety of approaches to the person, we may be able to clarify our own set of beliefs. It is only through clarifying what we believe that we can hope to change or modify our practice. What follows, then, is a brief exploration of some psychological approaches to counselling. Some will seem to be congruent with what we believe ourselves. Others will seem quite alien. The skill may be to try to adopt the psychological approach least like our own and to suspend judgement on it for a while. In trying out a new set of ideas in this way, we are already developing a skill that is vital in the process of counselling – that of adopting a frame of reference different from our own.

There is also a practical reason for adopting this approach. As we sit with a client, reflecting upon what they say in terms of the belief system we have about the nature of persons, so they too sit with their own belief system about the nature of the person. Clearly, there is no reason to suppose that the client's belief system, however hazy or well articulated, will correspond to our own. We cannot guarantee that the client has the same set of views about human nature as we do.

It is important, then, to consider a range of ways of making sense of human beings and of allowing theory to inform our practice. What follows does not claim to be an exhaustive classification of all possible views of the person but it will allow the individual reader to draw their own conclusions about why people may do the things they do and how best to help them in the counselling situation. The discussion here of the various approaches is necessarily brief and the reader is referred to the considerable literature on the topic for a more detailed exposition. The bibliography at the end of this book offers a variety of sources of further information.

THE PSYCHODYNAMIC APPROACH

Sigmund Freud is usually viewed as the father of the psychodynamic school of psychology (Hall, 1954). Essential to the approach is the notion that people are, to a greater or lesser extent, affected by unconscious motives and drives. That is to say, we cannot give a clear account of why we are behaving, thinking or feeling as we are, at any given time, because there are forces at work beneath the level of conscious awareness that cause us to act in a particular way. This unconscious level of the mind is developed out of experiences that happened to us in earlier parts of our lives that we were unable to deal with at the time. When we encounter an experience in the present that is in any way similar to that past event, we experience anxiety; we are unconsciously reminded of the situation.

For psychodynamic psychologists, then, the key to understanding a person's present behaviour is through a thorough exploration of their past. Thus, the psychodynamically oriented counsellor will usually choose to explore the client's past history and help them to identify and, if necessary, to relive various painful past events in order to make them less anxious and more able to make rational decisions about the present. In essence, then, the psychodynamic approach is a deterministic one. *Determinism* is the notion that every event has a cause and in this case, every aspect of a person's behaviour has a cause and that this cause is buried in the person's personal history. If you want to understand the person in the present, you must first understand their past. Essentially, too, a person's behaviour is basically understandable once these links to the past have been made. The process of counselling from the psychodynamic point of view may be likened to a jigsaw. Once all the pieces are put together, the whole thing makes sense. It is notable that many health professionals, particularly those in social work and certain types of nursing, may have been 'brought up' on the psychodynamic way of understanding people. It may be useful for them to explore other ways.

The psychodynamic approach has come under considerable criticism in recent years (Masson, 1990, 1992). In particular, Masson, in his study of Freud's archives, came to question Freud's 'seduction theory'. In early writings, Freud took the view that many women imagined that they had been sexually assaulted as children. Masson believes that Freud realized, later in his career, that many women were assaulted but his view that these memories were 'fantasies' was never corrected in classic psychoanalytical theory. In questioning classic theory in this way, Masson found himself out of favour with the psychoanalytical movement and subsequently gave up psychotherapy and counselling. An important lesson for counsellors in all this would seem to be that clients should, first of all, be believed. Given the levels of child abuse that have been 'discovered' in recent years, this is particularly important.

'Psychological mindedness' is described by Coltart (1993) as crucial if clients are to make use of psychoanalytic psychotherapy. If it is necessary for clients using this model, it must also be required of their therapists. Coltart lists nine qualities that she suggests add up to psychological mindedness, which she looks for when assessing patients for psychotherapy.

1 An acknowledgement, tacit or explicit, by the patient that they have an unconscious mental life and that it affects their thoughts and behavior.
2 The capacity to give a self-aware history, not necessarily in chronological order.
3 The capacity to give their history without prompting from the assessor and with some sense of the patient's emotional relatedness to the events of their own life and their meaning for them.
4 The capacity to recall memories, with the appropriate affects.
5 Some capacity to take the occasional step back from their own story and to reflect upon it, often with the help of a brief discussion with the assessor.
6 Signs of willingness to take responsibility for themselves and their own personal evolution.
7 Imagination, as expressed in imagery, metaphors, dreams, identifications with other people, empathy and so on.
8 Some signs of hope and realistic self-esteem. This may be faint, especially if the patient is depressed, but it is nevertheless important.
9 The overall impression of the development of the relationship with the assessor.

The psychodynamic approach in practice

The health professional who adopts the psychodynamic approach to counselling will tend to:

1 highlight the relationship between past and present life events;
2 acknowledge that unconscious forces are at work that affect the client's behaviour;
3 encourage the expression of pent-up emotion.

Examples of practical applications of this approach in the health care field include:

1 helping with long-term emotional problems;
2 coping with anxiety;
3 helping the client who talks of having had an unhappy childhood

THE COGNITIVE-BEHAVIOURAL APPROACH

While Freud was developing his theories in Europe around the turn of the century, John Watson in the USA was developing a different and opposing view of the person (Murphy and Kovach, 1972). He was adamant that the study of the person should be a scientific enterprise. To that end, he felt it should abandon the introspective methods suggested by Freud and concentrate on the arguably more objective study of human behaviour. Developing this theme, Watson argued that all human behaviour was learned and therefore could, if necessary, be unlearned. Such learning took place through the process he called *positive reinforcement*. Essentially, we learn those behaviours that we get encouraged to learn and forget those behaviours for which no encouragement is forthcoming. For the behavioural counsellor, then, the important issue is not the recollection of painful past events but the identification of what the client sees as undesirable behaviour. Once those undesirable (or uncomfortable) behaviours have been identified, the next step is to organize a scheme whereby more positive behaviours will be encouraged (or, in behavioural terms, a 'schedule of reinforcement' is drawn up). The client is then encouraged to go away and work at developing the desired behaviours through the scheme organized with the counsellor. No attempt is made to understand the cause of behaviours in terms of the past as no such theory of causation is mooted.

The behavioural approach may be described as a *mechanistic* approach in that it tends to view the person as a highly complex machine, perhaps rather like a computer. And just as a computer responds only to its programming, so the person responds only to the learning they have achieved through reinforcement. The key issues in the behavioural approach, then, are learning, unlearning and relearning. The behavioural approach is frequently used as the basis for the training of psychiatric nurse therapists.

Mehrabian (1971) highlights some of the advantages to this approach thus.

> *If we can find a way to expand the statement of a problem to a concrete list of specific behaviours which constitute it, one major obstacle to the solution of the problem will have been overcome. In other words, the initial ambiguity with which most people analyse their interpersonal problems tends to contribute to their feeling of helplessness in coping with them. Knowing which specific behaviours are involved, and thereby what changes in those behaviours will solve the problem, provides a definite goal for action – and having that goal can lead to a great sense of relief.*

Further, two other writers in the field indicate how important changes in behaviour are in helping people to change their perceptions of their situation.

> *Much of what we view clinically as 'abnormal behaviour' or 'emotional disturbance' may be viewed as ineffective behaviour and its*

consequences, in which the individual is unable to resolve certain situational problems in his life and his inadequate attempts to do so are having undesirable effects, such as anxiety, depression, and the creation of additional problems. (D'Zurilla and Goldfried, 1971)

In recent years, the strict form of behaviourism, with its insistence on the primacy of behaviour as a matter for scientific investigation, has given way to the *cognitive-behavioural approach*, with its accent on the fact that the way we *think* also affects our behaviour.

The cognitive-behavioural approach to counselling takes the view that what we think about ourselves affects the way we feel about ourselves. Thus, if we change our way of thinking, we can modify our feelings. Further, the argument is that many people hold exaggerated or incorrect beliefs about themselves that nevertheless affect their self-image. Examples of such false beliefs include 'No-one likes me', 'Everyone thinks I'm stupid' and 'I can't cope with anything'. These 'globalisms' or very general statements can have a negative effect on the person's functioning; the aim of the cognitive counsellor is to challenge these inaccurate and negative statements in order to modify the way the person thinks about himself and thus how he feels about himself.

Albert Ellis (1962), who developed 'rational emotive therapy', a particular sort of cognitive therapy, argued that there were 12 typical irrational beliefs that people could hold about themselves. They were not intended to be an exhaustive list of all possible irrational beliefs but represent commonly held erroneous beliefs that may have a profound effect on how a person thinks, feels and acts. The 12 beliefs that Ellis identified are:

1. It is a dire necessity that I be loved or approved of by everyone for everything I do.
2. Certain acts are wrong and evil and those who perform these acts should be severely punished.
3. It is terrible, horrible and catastrophic when things are not the way I would like them to be.
4. Unhappiness is caused by external events – it is forced upon one by external events, other people and circumstances.
5. If something is or may be dangerous or fearsome, I should be terribly concerned about it.
6. It is easier to avoid or replace life's difficulties than to face up to them.
7. I need someone or something stronger or greater than myself upon which I can rely.
8. I should be thoroughly competent, adequate and achieving in all the things I do and should be recognized as such.
9. Because something in my past strongly affected my life, it should indefinitely affect it.
10. What people do is vitally important to my existence and I should therefore make great efforts to change them to be more like the people I want them to be.

11 Human happiness can be achieved by inertia and inaction.
12 I have virtually no control over my emotions and I just cannot help feeling certain things.

Ellis claimed that anyone who holds any one or more of these beliefs is likely to experience distress inasmuch as they affect the way that person acts on those beliefs. Clearly this is a contentious list, but it is interesting and perhaps salutary to reflect on it and on the degree to which we ourselves hold any of these beliefs!

In the cognitive-behavioural approach, the style of counselling is one of challenging and confronting the client's belief system. In this respect, it is almost diametrically opposed to the style of counselling advocated by Carl Rogers – the client-centred approach. In the latter, the aim is to fully accept whatever the client says as a valid point of view about how that person views the world at that time. In the former approach, the aim is to call into question any number of beliefs that may be stopping the client from living fully and effectively. The approach has been used effectively with people who suffer from depression and other debilitating problems in living and practical examples of how the approach is used in practice are well described by Beck *et al.* (1979).

Technique and methods of cognitive-behavioural counselling

John Mcleod offers a useful list of the approaches used by some cognitive-behavioural counsellors.

1 Establishing rapport and creating a working alliance between counsellor and client. Explaining the rationale for treatment.
2 Assessing the problem. Identifying and quantifying the frequency, intensity and appropriateness of problem behaviours and cognitions.
3 Setting goals or targets for change. These should be selected by the client and be clear, specific and attainable.
4 Application of cognitive and behavioural techniques.
5 Monitoring progress, using ongoing assessment of target behaviours.
6 Termination and planned follow-up to reinforce generalization of gains.

He also suggests that the following techniques are commonly used.

- Challenging irrational beliefs.
- Reframing the issues: for example, perceiving internal emotional states as excitement rather than fear.
- Rehearsing the use for different self-statements in role plays with the counsellor.
- Experimenting with the use of different self-statements in real situations.

- Scaling feelings: for example, placing present feelings of anxiety or panic on a scale of 0–100.
- Thought stopping: rather than allowing anxious or obsessional thoughts to 'take over', the client learns to do something to interrupt them, such as snapping a rubber band on their wrist.
- Systematic desensitization: the replacement of anxiety or fear responses by a learned relaxation response. The counsellor takes the client through a graded hierarchy of fear-eliciting situations.
- Assertiveness or social skills training.
- Homework assignments: practising new behaviours and cognitive strategies between therapy sessions.
- *In vivo* exposure: being accompanied by the counsellor into highly fearful situations; for example, visiting shops with an agoraphobic client.

The cognitive-behavioural approach in practice

The health professional who adopts the cognitive behavioural approach to counselling will tend to:

1. rely less on personal warmth and more on confrontation in the counselling relationship;
2. use a logical and rational approach to problem solving;
3. encourage the client to develop a realistic and pragmatic outlook on life.

Examples of practical applications of this approach in the health-care field include:

1. helping the person who is depressed;
2. helping the person who has multiple problems;
3. encouraging rational thinking in someone who is highly emotional;
4. working with the person who has extreme anxiety by helping them to 'reframe' the emotion and to experience it as something else, such as excitement.

THE HUMANISTIC APPROACH

In the late 1940s and 1950s and perhaps reaching a peak in the 1960s, a movement began in psychology in America that challenged the determinism of psychodynamic psychology and the mechanism of behavioural psychology (Shaffer, 1978). This was what came to be known as the 'third force' in psychology – humanistic psychology. Drawing heavily on the field of existential philosophy, humanistic psychology argued that people were essentially free and responsible for their own condition. They were neither 'driven' by an unconscious mind nor were they only a product of what they had learned. Essentially, they were *agents*. The fact of consciousness gave them the ability to determine their own course of action through life and they were the best arbiters of what was and was not good for them. In humanistic psychology there could be no 'grand plan' of how people's minds work or how their behaviour could be manipulated. Humanistic psychology stressed individuality and individual differences in the human condition.

It was out of the humanistic school that the client-centred approach to counselling developed (Rogers, 1951). Rogers consistently argued that what made for effective counselling was trusting the individual's ability to find his own way through his problems. To this end, Rogers believed that people were essentially life-asserting and 'good', by nature. In this respect, he drew from the philosopher Rousseau and, perhaps more directly, from the American pragmatist and philosopher of science, John Dewey (1966, 1971). The aim of counselling for Rogers, then, was not necessarily to explore the person's past nor to necessarily try to modify their behaviour but to accept them and help them progress through their difficulties by their own route. Counsellors, then, were not experts in other people's problems but individuals who accompanied other people on their search for personal meaning. The client-centred approach has been pervasive in the counselling world; it has been adopted as a starting point for many training courses for counsellors and used in a variety of contexts in the health professions in the UK, from psychiatric nurse training (ENB, 1982) to the training of marriage guidance counsellors (MGC, 1983).

Arguably, it is out of the humanistic school of psychology that many of the 'alternative' counselling and therapy styles have arisen. A number of reasons for this development may be advanced. First, the humanistic school is an intensely *optimistic* one: it offers the individual the chance to take control of their life and does not posit the need to spend years of soul searching in order to do that. Second, historically, the humanistic school has developed alongside other changes in attitudes towards schooling and

The humanistic approach in practice

The health professional who adopts the humanistic approach to counselling will tend to:

1 avoid 'interpreting' the client's behaviour;
2 seek to encourage the client to identify his own solutions to his problems;
3 acknowledge that every individual is to some degree responsible for their own behaviour.

Examples of practical applications of this approach in the health care field include:

1 dealing with spiritual distress and problems of meaning;
2 helping with problems of self-image;
3 helping to free the client who believes that he is somehow controlled by his circumstances.

health care in both the USA and the UK. It seems almost inevitable that the humanistic approach would gradually find more popular acceptance amongst the 'new age' forms of therapy. Third (and this is by no means an exhaustive list), the methods used in the humanistic approach are relatively easy to learn and to put into practice. There is not a huge body of knowledge to absorb, as is the case with the psychodynamic approach, nor are there very particular skills to be learned, as is the case with the cognitive-behavioural approach. This latter point may also be one of criticism. Sometimes, the methods put forward under the heading of humanistic psychology are so vague or so abstract that it would be very difficult to assess the degree to which they are or are not effective.

THE TRANSACTIONAL ANALYSIS APPROACH

Transactional analysis may be described as a neo-Freudian approach to therapy.

Transactional analysis offers an economical way of describing and discussing people's relationships with one another. Formulated by the American psychotherapist, Eric Berne (1964, 1972), the analysis suggests that we all relate to other people (and the world) from three distinct 'ego states', described as the Parent, the Adult and the Child. When we operate from the Parent (which is developed through the early absorption of parental and judgemental attitudes), we tend to talk down to others, feel superior to them or patronize them. On the other hand, when we operate from the Child (which is mainly developed through our experiences of being a child), we tend to adopt a subservient relationship *vis-à-vis* other people. Thus, we become dependent upon them or submit too readily to their demands and feel uncomfortable as a result. Berne argues that the most appropriate method of relating to others is through the Adult, which is to say that we meet others as mature, equal beings.

Beyond this first formulation, it is possible to map the ways in which

The transactional analysis approach in practice

The health professional who adopts the transactional analysis approach to counselling will tend to:

1. notice the interpersonal 'games' that people play;
2. encourage the client to remain Adult in his relationships;
3. encourage the client to try new strategies in his relationships.

Examples of practical applications of this approach in the health care field include:

1. marital and relationship difficulties;
2. encouraging the client to become more assertive;
3. identifying more adult ways of dealing with problems.

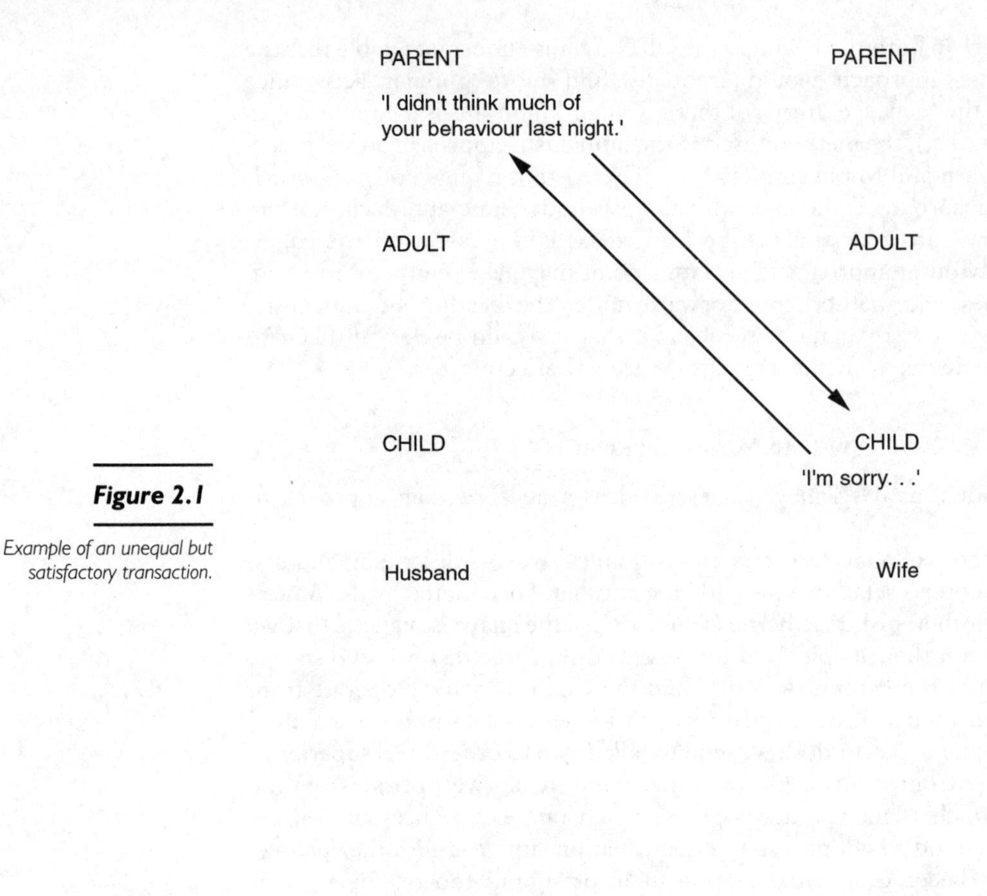

Figure 2.1

Example of an unequal but satisfactory transaction.

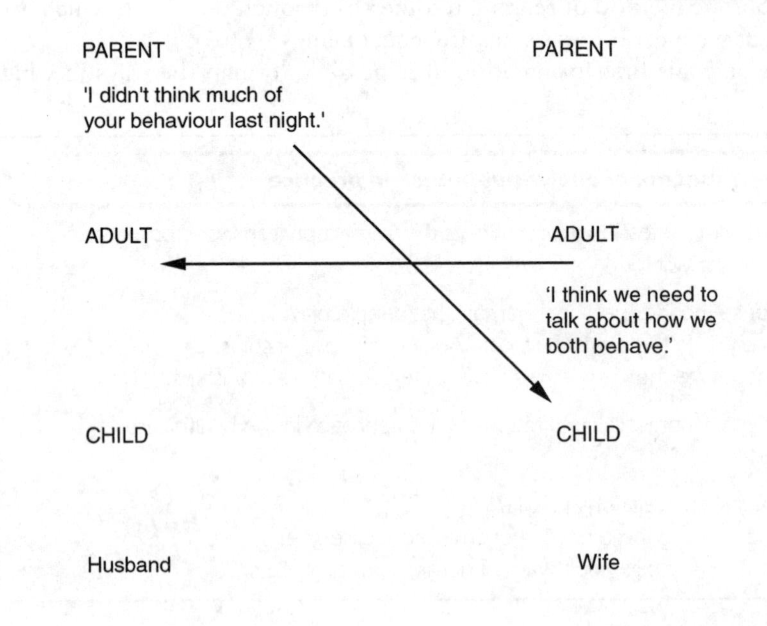

Figure 2.2

Example of an unequal and unsatisfactory transaction.

people relate to one another from ego state to ego state. Thus, a husband, for example, may relate to his wife from his Adult to her Child. Now if she is satisfied with this relationship, all well and good. Problems start, however, when the wife tries to relate to her husband on an Adult–Adult basis! This represents what Berne calls a 'crossed transaction' and will tend to lead to problems in the relationship (see Figures 2.1 and 2.2). The aim of transactional analysis is to enable clients to identify the sorts of relationship 'games' that they play with one another via these ego states and to learn more readily on an Adult–Adult basis.

THE PERSONAL-CONSTRUCT APPROACH

The personal-construct approach was developed by George Kelly (1955). Kelly used the metaphor of the scientist to describe how the person progresses through life. Thus, we predict how things will be in the near future (we develop a hypothesis). Then we test out that hypothesis in terms of what actually happens. As a result of what happens, we either consider our hypothesis confirmed or we discard it in favour of a revised hypothesis. Thus, according to Kelly, life is a series of personal predictions and confirmations or reconstructions. Our view of the world and of ourselves changes according to what happens to us and the sense we make of what happens to us.

Second, argues Kelly, we tend to view the world through a series of 'constructs' or 'ways of viewing' that colour our vision of how the world is. These constructs may be likened to different pairs of goggles that we put on at various times in order to make sense of what we perceive. An important point, here, is that the 'goggles' that we wear are not inaccurate or accurate or right or wrong; they merely represent different aspects of the world that stand out or are important for us.

Kelly devised an interesting way of exploring people's personal constructs and the following activity demonstrates how such constructs or ways of seeing can be elicited. Try the exercise now.

An exercise to explore personal constructs

Think of three people that you know. Choose people from different aspects of your life. You may, for example, choose (a) someone you live with, (b) someone you know at work and (c) a close friend, though any three people will be fine. Now consider a way in which two of those people are similar to each other and different from the third. This quality, behaviour or characteristic is what Kelly would call a *construct*. Now consider what you take to be the opposite of that quality, behaviour or characteristic. There are no right or wrong answers, but Kelly considers that this opposite characteristic represents another aspect of a person's construct system. Now consider to what degree you tend to view other people in terms of those two qualities, behaviours or characteristics.

You may like to try the activity again with a different trio of people and see what constructs you elicit in this case. If the process is repeated a number of times, you will tend to see a pattern of responses emerging. For Kelly, these represent something of your particular and idiosyncratic way of viewing the world.

It is important to say that no-one can interpret anything from your responses but they may give you some clarification as to what stands out about other people in your life experience.

For Kelly, then, the process of counselling can concern itself with exploring the ways in which the client construes the world around him. Gradually, through such exploration, the person can come to modify or change their construct system in order to make their lives more liveable.

Personal-construct psychology views the person as an evolving, dynamic subject who is continuously modifying his view of the world in the light of what happens to him. Thus, as we have seen, that person may be likened to a scientist and the person's constructs as the set of criteria, rules or methods of interpretation through which that person modifies or changes his picture of the world. Epting (1984) and Stewart and Stewart (1981) offer practical methods of using the personal-construct approach in counselling.

The personal-construct approach in practice

The health professional who adopts the personal-construct approach to counselling will tend to:

1. acknowledge that people differ from one another in fundamental ways;
2. look for the client's belief and value system as a clue to problem solving;
3. avoid interpreting the client's problem.

Examples of practical applications of this approach in the health-care field include:

1. helping the client to enhance self-awareness;
2. coping with marital and relationship difficulties;
3. 'unpacking' complex and multifaceted problems.

THE GESTALT-THERAPY APPROACH

The gestalt approach (it is usually spelt with a lower case 'g', perhaps to distinguish it from Gestalt psychology – a different thing altogether!) was devised by Fritz Perls (1969) who drew from a number of influences, including psychoanalysis, phenomenology, existentialism and Eastern philosophy (Smith, 1976). The German world *gestalt* is not easily translatable but roughly corresponds to the notion of wholeness or completeness.

The gestalt approach emphasizes the interplay between psychological or mental state and the state of the body, thus pointing up the totality of personal experience. It also concentrates on the changing and fluctuating nature of mental and physical state and concentrates most particularly on what is happening to the person now. It argues, reasonably, that the past is past and the future unknowable, therefore the focus of counselling attention should be the present moment. Thus, the gestalt approach encourages the client to become aware of what they are thinking, feeling and sensing, physically, in the here-and-now and how they restrict or limit themselves by making continuous reference to the past or how things may be in the future. Further, it uses a particular set of sometimes startling interventions to enable the client to explore various aspects of what is happening to them. As with the personal-construct and humanistic approaches, the emphasis is on the client interpreting or making sense of what is happening to them: it is not the counsellor's place to do that. The following dialogue may give something of the unique flavour of the gestalt approach.

Counsellor: What are you feeling at the moment?
Client: Nervous, odd.
Counsellor: Where in terms of your body do you feel that nervousness, oddness?
Client: (rubs his stomach)
Counsellor: Can you increase those feelings?
Client: Yes, but what a strange thing to ask! Yes, they're spreading up into my chest.
Counsellor: And what are you feeling now?
Client: It's changing . . . I'm feeling angry now!
Counsellor: Who are you angry with?
Client: Me! I realize that I've been bottling up my feelings for months!
Counsellor: OK . . . Just imagine that your bottled-up feelings are sitting in that chair over there . . . what do you want to say to them?
Client: Go away! You stop me getting on with what I want to do!
Counsellor: And what do the feelings say back to you?
Client: I keep you in check! I stop you from getting too involved with people!
Counsellor: And what do you make of all that?
Client: How odd! I realize how much I restrict myself by holding on to everything – it's becoming convenient! I feel different again, now . . . something else is happening.

And so the dialogue continues. The counsellor's aim is to stay with the client's moment-to-moment phenomenology or perception of himself and to help him to explore it. As we have noted, the counsellor does not interpret what the client says or offer suggestions as to how he may 'put his life right'. These are important principles in this person-centred and present-centred approach. Perls *et al.* (1951) offer a manual that, besides outlining the principles and theory of the gestalt approach, suggests a wide range of do-it-yourself gestalt exercises to increase self-awareness and clarify perception. A number of colleges and extra-mural departments of universities in both the UK and the USA offer short and extended courses in the gestalt approach.

The gestalt-therapy approach in practice

The health professional who adopts the gestalt-therapy approach to counselling will tend to:

1 treat each counselling situation as unique;
2 deal with issues as they arise and in the here-and-now;
3 notice small, non-verbal behaviours exhibited by the client.

Examples of practical applications of this approach in the health-care field include:

1 helping the client who bottles up emotion;
2 helping the person who has difficulty in verbalizing his problems;
3 coping with problems of self-image and self-confidence.

WHICH IS THE MAIN APPROACH USED TODAY?

The answer to this does, of course, depend on where you are standing and on your particular point of view. In general terms, though, there is a tendency towards counsellors being able to *demonstrate* that what they do is effective. In the 'purchaser–provider' climate of the new health care service in the UK, this demand for evidence-based practice is likely to become more acute. To this end, there is evidence that, currently, the cognitive-behavioural approach to counselling is becoming more popular, perhaps at the expense of the psychodynamic approach. The humanistic approach remains popular given the fact that its methods are relatively easy to teach and learn and perhaps because, historically, they have been used for so long. It seems that the emphasis will continue to be on establishing forms of counselling that are economical, able to be practised over a relatively short space of time and which can be demonstrated to be effective. At the time of writing, the counselling approach that seems most likely to meet these criteria is the cognitive-behavioural approach or a variant of it.

THE ECLECTIC APPROACH

In the end, what we do in counselling depends upon a number of issues: our skill levels, what we feel comfortable doing in the counselling relationship, our belief and value systems as they relate to how we view what people are 'about', our level of self-awareness, our mood at the time, our present life situation, our perception of what (if anything) is wrong with the client, current work load and time available and many other factors. Thus, it is reasonable to argue that no one set of counselling tools or no one particular approach can be appropriate in every counselling situation. It is perhaps more useful if the health professional considers a wide range of possibilities, tries out some of the approaches (first, perhaps, with a willing colleague and in return, having that colleague try them out on the health professional!) and slowly incorporates the approaches that most suit that person into a personal repertoire. This personal repertoire or personal style offers the most flexible approach to counselling – the eclectic approach. Further, it is in line with Heron's argument in Chapter 1 (p. 27) that the counsellor becomes skilled in a wide range of possible counselling interventions in order to help a wide range of people. After all, health professionals meet a wide range of clients varying considerably in their cultural backgrounds, their personal experience, belief systems, needs, wants and wishes, political persuasions and personal psychologies. It is important that we offer clients what they want and not necessarily what we perceive that they need. The counselling relationship belongs to the client and not to the counsellor: we should not be dazzling them with a range of counselling interventions but finding out what they really want. In a sense, this is almost overwhelmingly simple for as Epting notes, echoing the social psychologists Allport, Kelly and others: 'If you want to know what someone is about, ask them – they may just tell you!' (Epting, 1984).

The eclectic approach in practice

The health professional who adopts the eclectic approach to counselling will tend to:

1 believe that no one approach to counselling suits each situation;
2 read widely and learn a variety of different sorts of counselling skills;
3 run the risk of being 'jack of all counselling skills and master of none'!

Examples of practical applications of this approach in the health-care field include:

1 everyday counselling practice;
2 working with the client who does not respond to a particular counselling approach;
3 helping the person who has very varied problems in living.

IS IT POSSIBLE TO DO WITHOUT A THEORY OF THE PERSON?

In this chapter, we have reviewed various ways of thinking about how people 'work'. Is it possible, then, to do counselling without any particular theory of the person? In the strict sense, probably not. The very fact that we choose to say 'I do not have any particular theories about human beings' is a theoretical stance in itself. However, I believe that it is possible to manage with *minimal* theory, especially as all the above theories are, to a greater or lesser extent, empirically untested. It would be difficult to state, once and for all, that one theory approaches 'the truth' more nearly than another – although, arguably, some theories are more open to testing than others.

However, we can take the view that, as people vary widely and as it is impossible to completely understand other people's minds, then we can use theory parsimoniously in our work as counsellors. To this end, I would like to suggest the following principles for reflection and discussion.

- It may be best not to make any particular assumptions about *why* the person in front of us does the things that they do.
- It may be best to *believe* what the other person says to us – at least until they contradict themselves or indicate otherwise.
- The person in front of us may be similar to us or very different from us and we should, not make any assumptions about those similarities or differences.
- It is possible that people do things *for no particular reason at all*. This, too, is important in counselling.
- It seems probable that some people find talking about their problems useful and that some people do not.
- It may or may not be true that past experiences influence the way we are today. It is also possible that some people are more affected by their past than others. The *importance* of recalling the past and linking it to present-day events and actions has not yet been proven.
- Given that memories are often faulty, it may be better to be *future focused* rather than focused on trying to work out why any given person is the way that they are. After all, we live our lives forward.

Herein lies the paradox: the above statements could be construed as the beginning of a theory! My point, though, is that we need to theorize about other people as little as possible, to listen to them, to focus on the future and to worry less about the 'why' than the 'what comes next'. It is, if you like, a pragmatic approach to counselling.

PSYCHOLOGICAL APPROACHES TO COUNSELLING AND THE HEALTH PROFESSIONAL

As we have noted, no one school of psychology or theoretical approach to counselling offers *the* way of viewing the person. The approaches offer different ways of looking at the person which are not necessarily mutually exclusive. Which of the approaches the health professional chooses to use as a guide to understanding the process of counselling will depend on a number of factors, including, at least: their original psychological training that accompanied their basic professional training, the influences of any workshops, study days or further training, exposure to colleagues and friends who offer different points of view, further reading around the topic and so forth.

Another deciding factor may be the type of relationship that the health professional has with the client and the amount of time they spend together. The social worker, the speech therapist and the psychiatric nurse may all spend considerable time building up a relationship that, itself, may last for months or even years. On the other hand, the physiotherapist and the occupational therapist may have a shorter if quite intense relationship. It may be that the shorter relationships require a pragmatic psychology that allows for goals to be set and achieved; in this sense, the behavioural approach offers usable concepts that can help to structure the relationship. If a longer term relationship is being developed, a 'process' model may be more applicable and the health-professional-as-counsellor may wish to consider those models that emphasize the quality of the relationship and an analysis of what is going on in that relationship. Here, the psychodynamic and humanistic approaches may help. In the end, the psychological model adopted for understanding the counselling relationship will depend on the health professional's own beliefs about the nature of people. In order to clarify what our beliefs are, we need to develop a degree of self-awareness – the topic of the following chapter.

We have also noted in this chapter that the health care climate is changing – at least in the UK – towards the need for *evidence-based practice* and the need for counsellors and those who use counselling skills to *demonstrate* that what they do is effective.

3 Counselling and Self-Awareness

It would seem reasonable to say that if we are to help others, we should first know something of ourselves. Self-awareness is an essential component in the counselling process. It is necessary for a number of reasons, which will be discussed first before the questions of self-awareness itself are addressed.

First, self-awareness allows us to discriminate between our own problems and those of the client. If we do not have at least a minimal self-awareness, it is easy for us to identify with the other person's problems and to imagine that they are similar to, or even the same as, our own. The reverse of this situation is also possible. Without self-awareness, it is possible to imagine that everyone else (and particularly this client) has the same problems as we do. In this way, our own problems are projected onto the client. We need to be able to identify clear 'ego boundaries': to make a clear distinction between ourselves and our client. As a matter of fact, what the client is describing at any particular time is never the same as a situation we have found ourselves in. It may be similar to it, but it can never be the same. Self-awareness helps us to mark out our ego boundaries and successfully discriminate between what belongs to us and what belongs to the client. Haydn (1965) describes the problem well when he writes:

> *Day by day, hour by hour, we misunderstand each other because we cross well-marked boundaries; we blur the sense of you out there and me here; we merge, frequently very sloppily, the subjective with the objective, in various ways. We make of the other person simply an extension of self, either through the attribution of our own thoughts and attitudes to the other person, or by too facile a decision about his nature, after which we go on responding to him as though he were the character we invented.*

Such demarcation is also an essential part of the counsellor taking care of herself. When ego boundaries become blurred, considerable emotion is invested in the relationship by the counsellor and the net result can be *burnout* – emotional and physical exhaustion as a result of work-related stress. Burnout manifests itself in the following ways:

- disillusionment with the job;
- a feeling of hopelessness and inability to cope;
- a need to get away from people;
- a loss of ability to empathize with others.

Burnout can be prevented through reflection on our performance and through developing self-awareness, as discussed below.

Second, self-awareness enables us to make what Heron (1977b) calls 'conscious use of the self'. Without awareness we will tend to feel that any counselling interventions we make are spontaneous and not offered consciously. Now, the point of conscious use of the self is that we learn to reflect on what is happening during the counselling relationship and we choose the interventions we make. In other words, the words and phrases that we use are intended and chosen consciously, rather than just happening. Initially, such conscious use of the self can seem awkward and clumsy. We tend to be socialized into dividing human action up into natural (and therefore, presumably, sincere) and contrived (and therefore, presumably, insincere). The suggestion that we choose particular types of words or expressions smacks of unnaturalness and therefore tends to sound disagreeable.

On reflection, however, it may be noted that all other human skills, apart from listening and talking to others, are learned through the process of consciously considering what we are doing. If we are to become skilled as nurses, doctors or social workers, we must concentrate on what we do and observe the outcomes of our actions. The verbal skills of counselling can also be learned in a similar way and the concept of 'conscious use of self' has a variety of applications.

As we have already noted, in the first place, such use of the self can enable us to choose the right sort of counselling intervention for the right occasion. It can bring clarity and precision to the counselling relationship. If, for example, we use the category analysis identified in the previous chapter, we can vary our repertoire of verbal interventions in a way that helps this particular person at this particular time. In this sense, then, the conscious use of the self enhances sensitivity to the other person's needs.

Next, conscious use of the self can help us to distinguish between the client's problems and our own. In this way it serves to maintain and clarify the ego boundaries alluded to at the beginning of this chapter. In the process of developing conscious use of the self, we learn to notice ourselves and to pay attention to how we are reacting to the unfolding counselling session. Such self-noticing can enable us, again, to make more sensitive use of our counselling interventions, to be more tactful and truly meet the arising needs of the client. This process also has other connotations, for as Rollo May (1983) notes, what the counsellor is feeling is often a direct reflection of what the client is feeling, once the counselling relationship deepens and becomes more intense. Thus, attention by the counsellor to her own changing feelings can help in the process of understanding and empathizing with the client.

The process of developing conscious use of self can be uncomfortable. Three stages in its development may be noted and these are described below.

First stage

In this stage, the person is unaware of the range of possible skills and interventions that are available to them. This is the stage of being natural or spontaneous. There is a tendency, in this stage, for the person to believe that people are 'born counsellors' and that the skills of counselling either come naturally to the individual or they cannot be developed at all. This may be called the unskilled stage.

Second stage

In the second stage of the process, the person becomes aware of the possible range of interventions available and feels clumsy as a result. This may be compared to the process of learning to drive a car. In the first place, we do not know how to drive the car at all. As we learn to drive, we have to pay attention to a wide range of different actions and the net result is that we are awkward and clumsy. So it is with the process of learning counselling through conscious use of the self. This may be called the clumsy stage.

Third stage

In the final stage of learning, the interventions involved in counselling are absorbed by the person and they become skilled. Conscious use of the self has become a normal part of their repertoire of behaviour and no longer feels awkward or clumsy. Interestingly, too, the naturalness returns. The skills, having been learned, emerge without forethought; the counsellor no longer has to consider what to say or what not to say but readily responds in the counselling situation out of the wide range of skills that have become her own. What remains conscious, however, is the ability to notice what is happening as the relationship unfolds. What has changed is the ability to act in an appropriate and sensitive manner whilst being guided by the observations made during this process of noticing. This may be called the skilled stage of counselling development.

NOTICING IN THE DEVELOPMENT OF COUNSELLING SKILLS

It will be noted that frequent reference is made to the notion of *noticing*, of paying close attention to what is happening both in the counselling relationship and in the counsellor herself. This notion is central to the whole process of learning to become a skilful and effective counsellor. It is also a central concept in the idea of self-awareness and one that will be referred to again in this context. Clearly, unless we notice what is happening to us, we cannot become self-aware. In exploring the notion of self-awareness as it applies to counselling, it will be useful, first, to consider the concept of the self.

The action of noticing can be readily used in any health care setting. It is useful and instructive merely to notice our reactions to certain situations. For instance, consider your reactions to any of the following:

- attempted suicide;
- severe incontinence in a young adult;
- severe and disfiguring handicap;
- the psychiatric patient admitted to a general ward.

We may want to argue that, as professionals, we do not react to such human problems but we take action to help them. If this sort of argument is offered, it is worth listening a little closer to what is going on inside! It is easy for us to delude ourselves that we do not react to extreme aspects of human suffering as do other non-professionals. Again, it is salutary to question this stance and vital to do so if we are to become effective counsellors. We can never afford to become 'case hardened' as carers or as counsellors.

THE SELF

The idea of what it means to have a self has been discussed down through the ages by philosophers, theologians, psychologists, sociologists, psychiatrists and political theorists. Psychologists have approached the concept from many points of view. Some have tried to analyse the factors that make up the self, rather as a chemist might try to discover the chemicals that are present in a particular solution. Others have argued that there are certain consistent aspects of the self that determine, to some extent, the way in which we live our lives. Psychoanalytical theory, as we have seen, argues that early childhood experiences profoundly affect and shape the self, determining how we react to the world as adults. Childhood experiences, in this theoretical construction, lay the foundations of the self that may be modified by life experience but, nevertheless, stay with us throughout life. Such a view, as we noted earlier, is deterministic in that it argues that our present sense of self is determined by earlier life experiences and we are shaped, to a greater or lesser extent, by our childhood.

Other psychological theorists argue that there are problems with reductionist theories – theories that attempt to analyse the self into discrete parts. Such theorists prefer to view the self from a holistic or gestalt perspective. This approach argues that the totality of the self is always something more than the sum of its parts. Just as we cannot discover exactly what we like about a piece of music by examining it note by note, neither can we fully understand the self by compartmentalizing it. In this sense, then, the self can never be completely defined, for the subject of our study – the self – is always evolving and is always more than the sum of its parts.

It is worth noting, too, that we do not exist as selves-in-isolation. What we are and who we are depends, to a very considerable extent, on the other people with whom we live, work and relate. Our sense of self also depends upon how those other people define us. In this sense, other people are frequently telling us who we are. As health professionals, we rely on other colleagues, on clients and on friends offering us both positive and negative feedback on our performance as people. Such feedback is slowly absorbed by the individual, modifying and (hopefully) enhancing the sense of self.

A note of caution is important. The idea of the self is an *abstraction*. It is a way of talking about inner aspects of the person. To this end, it cannot be said to 'exist', in the way that a table or a book exists. We should therefore be careful of at least two things. First is the temptation to *reify* the self.

Reification is the mistake of treating an abstraction as though it does have concrete reality and therefore making more dogmatic claims about it than are reasonable to make. Second is an awareness of the fact that when we talk about abstractions, we are basing our discourse on belief rather than on fact. You cannot, in the end, *demonstrate* aspects of the self. The following debate, then, is necessarily a tentative one and one that you may or may not agree with. What is probably more important, as a person using counselling skills, is for you to consider what *your* beliefs are about the nature of the self.

It may be useful, then, to consider the range of aspects that may go to make up a sense of self. As with any such analysis of self, it cannot be exhaustive but it may serve to highlight the complex and multifaceted nature of the subject. Five aspects of self are considered here:

1. the physical self;
2. the private self;
3. the social self;
4. the spiritual self;
5. the-self-as-defined-by-others.

Clearly, it would be impossible to capture all the facets implied by the term 'self'. The account that follows is a 'shorthand' way of considering aspects of the self as they apply to the field of counselling.

The physical self

The physical self refers to the bodily or 'felt' sense of self. We are all (like it or not!) contained within a body and our perception of what we and other people think we look like contributes to how we see ourselves as a person. Further, there is an intimate link between how we feel psychologically and how we feel physically. To argue otherwise is to invoke the famous Cartesian split – the notion (propounded by the French philosopher Descartes) that the body and the mind could be considered separately. The acknowledgement that the mind and body are so closely linked (and, arguably, the body 'produces' the mind) has considerable implications for counselling, as we shall see in later chapters. Suffice it to say, here, that in noticing our 'body self' we may learn much about how we perceive ourselves generally. Noticing changing bodily sensations can be one route towards developing self-awareness.

The private self

The private self alludes to that part of us that we live inside: the hidden part of us that we reveal slowly – if at all – to other people. R.D. Laing (1959) has written a considerable amount on this concept and suggested that it is quite possible for the 'private' self to watch the 'public' self in action! Certainly, from the point of view of developing self-awareness, it is useful to become aware of this inner, private self and to notice to what degree and with whom that private sense of self is shared. Again, from the counselling point of view, such a notion of private self has considerable relevance, for it is the private self that is often shared in the counselling relationship.

It is worth thinking about the degree to which there is a *gap* between private and public aspects of self. When you are particularly upset, disturbed or preoccupied, it may become 'safer' to present quite a different 'public' self to the self that is churning away beneath the surface. The question remains, however, to what degree a person with a completely 'hidden' sense of self can make an effective counsellor. After all, in counselling, the counsellor is inviting the client to share something of their private self with the counsellor. If, for their part, the counsellor is unable to share something of *their* private self, then the relationship becomes particularly unbalanced. Another view, of course, is that the counselling relationship is always unbalanced, for it is always the client who is expected to disclose aspects of themselves and no such disclosure is expected of the counsellor.

The social self

The social self is that aspect of the person that is shared openly with others. It may be contrasted with the private self. It is the self that we choose to show to other people. The degree to which there is congruence between our private self and our social self may indicate our level of emotional and interpersonal security. Both Rogers (1951) and Laing (1959) have argued that when there is a close correspondence between the inner experience of self and the outer presentation of it, emotional security and stability tend to be present also. It is interesting and salutary to reflect on the degree to which this is true for us at the moment of reading this! As we have noted above, a great discrepancy between the one and the other may indicate personal problems of a magnitude that make functioning as a counsellor difficult.

The spiritual self

The spiritual self refers to the aspect that is concerned with a search for personal meaning. As we noted in the first chapter, personal meaning may be framed within a variety of contexts: religious, philosophical, political, sociological, psychological and so forth. It is the spiritual aspect of the self that makes sense of what is happening to the person. It is that aspect of self concerned with belief and value systems. It may also be that part of the self that is concerned with the *transpersonal* aspects of being – that which unites all persons. Rogers (1967) has alluded to such a dimension when he concluded that what is most personal in the counselling relationship is, almost paradoxically, most universal.

Developing this notion of the transpersonal further, Jung (1978) argued for the existence of a 'collective unconscious' – a domain that contains all human experience, both past and present, to which we all have access. Supporting arguments for the existence of this collective unconscious include what Jung called synchronicity or meaningful coincidence. We may, for example, be thinking of someone and they phone us or we are about to say something and the person we are with says exactly the same thing. These are examples of synchronous events. The appearance of symbols in dreams is also offered as evidence for the collective unconscious: Jung maintained that certain types of symbols (crosses and circles, for example) occur through the ages in all parts of the world and in many contexts and cultures. Further, these symbols often appear in our dreams and Jung argues that such appearances are made possible through our tapping the collective unconscious. Jung did not offer the concept dogmatically but suggested that it may be useful in trying to make sense of those aspects of self that seem to be shared by all persons.

The self-as-defined-by-others

The self-as-defined-by-others refers to the way in which others see us. This is a particularly complicated issue in that how others see us will depend upon so many variables. Their perception of us will be coloured by at least the following factors: their relationship to us, their previous experiences of people who are like us and different from us, how they think we view them, their views on sexuality, race and roles, their own view of themselves. The matter is further complicated by the fact that other people's perception of us is, presumably, not static. It changes according to the aforementioned variables and in accordance with our relationship with them.

This issue of the self-as-defined-by-others is of particular importance in counselling. The client's view of the counsellor at any given time in the relationship may serve as a useful barometer for measuring the nature and depth of the relationship. At times, their view of the counsellor will be unequivocally positive; at others it will be far less so. All these changes reflect, to a greater or lesser degree, the amount of dependence and independence that the client is maintaining at that particular time. This changing concept of the counsellor in the eyes of the client has been called *transference* and is explored further in Chapter 9.

These, then, are some of the many facets that go to make up a sense of self. Another way of making sense of the concept of self is to view it in terms of different types of knowledge.

The self defined through types of knowledge

Three types of knowledge that go to make up an individual may be described: propositional knowledge, practical knowledge and experiential knowledge (Heron, 1981). Whilst each of these types is different, they are all inter-related. Thus, whilst propositional knowledge may be considered as qualitatively different from, say, practical knowledge, it is possible and probably better to use propositional knowledge in the application of practical knowledge.

Propositional knowledge

Propositional knowledge is knowledge that is contained in theories or models. It may be described as textbook knowledge and is synonymous with Ryle's (1949) concept of 'knowing that', which was developed further in an educational context by Pring (1976). Thus, a person may build up a considerable bank of facts, theories or ideas about a subject, person or thing, without necessarily having any direct experience of that subject, person or thing. A person may, for example, develop a considerable propositional knowledge about, say, midwifery without ever having been anywhere near a woman who is having a baby! Presumably, it would be more useful to combine that knowledge with some practical experience, but this does not necessarily have to be the case. This, then, is the domain of propositional knowledge. Obviously it is possible to have propositional knowledge about a great number of subject areas ranging from mathematics to literature or from counselling to social work. Any information contained in books (including this one!) must necessarily be of the propositional sort.

Practical knowledge

Practical knowledge is knowledge that is developed through the acquisition of skills. Thus, driving a car or giving an injection demonstrates practical knowledge, though, equally, so does the use of counselling skills that involve specific verbal and non-verbal behaviours and intentional use of counselling interventions. Practical knowledge is synonymous with Ryle's (1949) concept of 'knowing how', which was developed further in an educational context by Pring (1976). Usually more than a mere knack, practical knowledge is the substance of a smooth performance of a practical or interpersonal skill. A considerable amount of a health professional's time is taken up with the demonstration of practical knowledge – often, but not always, of the interpersonal sort.

Traditionally, most educational programmes in schools and colleges have concerned themselves primarily with both propositional and practical knowledge, particularly the former. Thus, the propositional knowledge aspect of a person is the aspect that is often held in highest regard. Practical knowledge, although respected, is usually seen as slightly less important. In this way, the self can become highly developed in one sense – the propositional knowledge aspect – at the expense of being skilled in a practical sense.

Experiential knowledge

Experiential knowledge is knowledge gained through direct encounter with a subject, person or thing. It is the subjective and affective nature of that encounter that contributes to this sort of knowledge. Experiential knowledge is knowledge through relationships. It is synonymous with Rogers' (1983) description of experiential learning and with Polanyi's (1958) concept of 'personal' knowledge and 'tacit' knowledge. If we reflect for a moment, we may discover that most of the things that are really important to us belong in this domain. If, for example, we consider our personal relationships with other people, we discover that what we like or love about them cannot be reduced to a series of propositional statements and yet the feelings we have for them are vital and part of what is most important in our lives. Most encounters with others contain the possible seeds of experiential knowledge. It is only when we are so detached from other people that we treat them as objects that no experiential learning can occur.

Not that all experiential learning is tied exclusively to relationships with other people. For example, I had considerable propositional knowledge about America before I went there. When I went there, all that propositional knowledge was changed considerably. What I had known was changed by my direct experience of the country. I had developed experiential knowledge of the place. Experiential knowledge is not of the same type or order as propositional or practical knowledge. It is, nevertheless, important knowledge, in that it affects everything else we think about or do.

Experiential knowledge is necessarily personal and idiosyncratic. Indeed, as Rogers (1985) points out, it may be difficult to convey to another person in words. Words tend to be loaded with personal (often experiential) meanings and thus to understand each other, we need to understand how the people with whom we converse use words. It is arguable, however, that such experiential knowledge is sometimes conveyed to others through gesture, eye contact, tone of voice, inflection and all the other non-verbal and paralinguistic aspects of communication (Argyle, 1975). Indeed, it may be experiential knowledge that is passed on when two people (for example, a counsellor and her client) become very involved with each other in a conversation, a learning encounter or counselling. Counselling, then, may be concerned very much with the discussion of experiential knowledge: certainly, it is more about this domain than it is about the domains of propositional or practical knowledge.

These three domains of knowledge are important aspects of a sense of self. What we know in these three domains is what we are. Thus, a balanced sense of self within this framework is achieved by a balance between our theoretical knowledge, what we can do with it in terms of practical and interpersonal skills and what we have in terms of personal experience. All three domains grow and increase throughout the life cycle, though they are not always equally recognized. As we have seen, propositional knowledge tends to take precedence over the other two and, in academic terms, experiential knowledge often counts for very little.

From the points of view of counselling and self-awareness, it may be useful to keep all three aspects in balance. The skilled counsellor, then, is one who combines theoretical knowledge about counselling with well-developed interpersonal competence and considerable life experience.

THE CONCEPT OF PERSONHOOD

Yet another way of considering the self is via the notion of *personhood*: what it means to be a person. If we can identify those basic criteria that distinguish persons from all other sorts of things, we may be clearer about what it means to talk of the self. Bannister and Fransella (1986) offer a list of criteria for personhood that may be helpful in clarifying such a notion. It is argued that you consider yourself a person in that:

1 you entertain a notion of your own separateness from others; you rely on the privacy of your own consciousness;
2 you entertain a notion of the integrality or completeness of your experience, so that you believe all parts of it are relatable because you are the experiencer;
3 you entertain a notion of your own continuity over time; you possess your own biography and live in relation to it;
4 you entertain a notion of the causality of your actions: you have purposes, you intend, you accept a partial responsibility for the effects of what you do;
5 you entertain a notion of other persons by analogy with yourself; you assume a comparability of subjective experience.

Such a notion of personhood can do much to clarify what it means to entertain a notion of self and may also serve as a framework for understanding the personal factors that we are addressing in the process of counselling. For if we accept Bannister and Fransella's idea of personhood, then we necessarily accept that idea as applying to the person who is in front of us in the counselling relationship. The notion of personhood addresses the concepts of separateness from others, completeness of human experience, personal biography, at least partial responsibility for actions and appreciation of other persons as being similar to ourselves. All these concepts are addressed when one person sets out to counsel another.

AN INTEGRATED MODEL OF THE SELF

What is needed now is a model that brings together the notions of self so far described. Figure 3.1 offers a fairly comprehensive model of the self through which to understand the idea of self-awareness. It incorporates Jung's work on the four functions of the mind: thinking, feeling, sensing and intuiting (Jung, 1978) and also an adaptation of Laing's (1959) concept of an inner and outer self. The outer, public self is what others see of us and is compatible with the notion of the self-as-defined-by-others, described on p. 56. The inner, private aspect is what goes on in our heads and bodies. In one sense, the outer experience is what other people are most familiar with. We communicate the inner experience through the outer. Our thoughts, feelings and experiences are all communicated through this outer experience of behaviour. Of what does it consist?

The outer experience of the self

At its most simple, behaviour consists of body movements, the crossing of arms and legs, walking, running and so forth. At a more subtle level, however, the issue becomes more complicated. There is a whole variety of more subtle behaviours that convey the inner sense of self through the outer. First, there is speech. The words, phrases, metaphors and expressions we use are a potent means by which we convey feelings, thoughts and experiences to others. How we come to choose these particular words, phrases

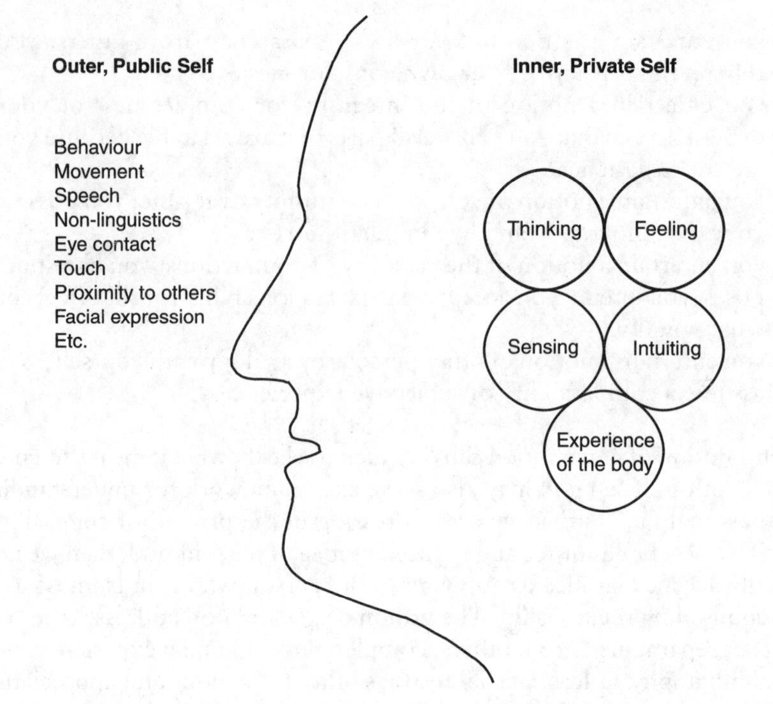

Figure 3.1

An integrated model of the self.

and expressions, however, depends upon many variables including our past experiences, our education, our cultural inheritance, our knowledge of the language, our attitudes, our belief systems, our social positions and the company we are in. Alongside those words and phrases are the non-linguistic aspects of speech, including timing, pitch, pacing, silences and so on. Such non-linguistic aspects of communication are subtle ways of communicating aspects of our inner selves to others.

When we talk to other people, we usually look at them. Heron (1970) notes that there can be wide variety in the intensity, amount and quality of eye contact. Our emotional status and our relationship with the person with whom we are speaking tend to govern the amount of eye contact we allow ourselves to make with them and the amount we expect in return. In the context of counselling, it is important to remain sensitive to aspects of eye contact and to consciously monitor the amount we use in relation to the client. Such monitoring of eye contact is in line with the notion of conscious use of the self, described on p. 51.

The amount of physical contact or touch that we have with others is also a potent means of conveying our inner experience to others. Typically, we touch those people to whom we are close more: members of the family, people we love and very close friends. Some people, it would seem, are 'high touchers' and others 'low touchers'. There are also cultural factors governing the use of touch between people of different races, between sexes and between people of different relative status. Again, in the context of counselling, we need to be careful that our use of touch is unambiguous, acceptable to the client and never viewed by that person as an intrusion. If we are a high toucher, for example, we cannot assume that all our clients are also high touchers!

When we relate to others, the fact of verbally communicating with them means that we necessarily are near them. How we sit or stand in relation to others is determined by a number of factors, including the level of intimacy we have with them, our relationship with them, certain cultural factors, personal preferences for closeness or lack of it and whether or not we occupy a dominant or subordinate position *vis-à-vis* the other person (Brown, 1986). In the counselling relationship, it is easy for the counsellor to forget that she is occupying a dominant position simply by being the counsellor! As a result, the temptation is sometimes to sit closer to the client than is comfortable for him. An easy, practical solution to this is to allow the client to draw up the chair and thus to define the personal space between counsellor and client.

Another indicator of our inner experience is our facial expression. Raised eyebrows, grins and sneers can do much to convey to others our internal states. An important concept, here, is that of *congruence* in communication. Bandler and Grinder (1975) identify three aspects of congruence. A person is said to be congruent when:

1 what they say, matches
2 how they say it and
3 both are matched by the appropriate facial expression.

If one or more of these factors does not match, then communication is likely to be unclear. Sometimes these mismatches are caused by internal conflicts or by our not saying what we really mean. In terms of counselling, it is important that we learn to be congruent in our dealings with others. We must be seen to mean what we say: just saying it is not sufficient! Such congruence needs careful attention and a considerable amount of self-awareness. It is surprising how easily ambiguous thoughts 'leak out' through our facial expressions! External congruence in terms of words, tone of voice and facial expression also calls for internal congruence in terms of being clear about what we think and feel about what we are saying. It is rare that we can completely disguise our internal thoughts and feelings and anyway, if we are to be genuine in our counselling, it is important that we be clear, honest and unambiguous.

These, then, are aspects of the outer self – that part of ourselves that others see and through which we communicate our inner experience. Not that such outer, visible behaviour is read entirely accurately by others. When other people perceive us, they do so through their own particular frame of reference and tend to interpret what they see in terms of that frame. No-one views another objectively. Everyone's perception of others is more or less coloured by their own history and experience. All the more reason, then, as counsellors to ensure that our external behaviour is as clear and as genuine as it can be. It will be misread by the client at times, but less so if our initial intentions are clear.

The inner experience of the self

The inner, private experience of the self may be divided into (a) aspects of mental function according to Jung's typography: thinking, feeling, sensing and intuiting; and (b) the experience of the body. As we have already noted, this division will necessarily be artificial as both mental and physical events are inextricably linked. As Searle (1983) acknowledges, a mental event is also a physical one. Physical status also affects mental and psychological performance and a person's self-concept. It is interesting to note the growing interest in healing this apparent split between the mind and the body. Increasingly, the move is towards a holistic approach in health care that emphasizes the inter-relatedness between mind, body and (sometimes) spirit. Any concept of self must take into account the mind and body as a totality.

Thinking

Thinking refers to all the aspects of our mental processes, both logical and illogical. If we reflect on thinking we will realize that it is not a linear process. We do not think in sentences or even in logical sequences of phrases. The whole process is much more haphazard than that and has much in common with the technique known as *free association*, used in psychoanalysis. Free association asks of the client that he repeats whatever comes into his mind. The result is usually a string of not obviously related statements, ideas and expressions of feelings. Such, perhaps, is the nature of thinking.

Nor can we be sure that our thinking is accurate or realistic. As we noted in the last chapter, Kelly (1955) argued that we are continually creating hypotheses about how the world is and then testing those hypotheses in the light of our experience. In this sense, then, thinking may be concerned with the creation of a number of theories about the world. Guy Claxton (1984) suggests an important pair of principles on this issue. He argues that:

1 what I do depends on what my theory tells me about the world, not on how the world really is; and
2 what happens next depends on how the world really is, not how I believe it to be.

Thus, if our theory about how the world is is very distorted, there will be a sense of jarring as we progress though it. If our theory about the world is grounded in some sort of reality, then our perception of the world and our place in it will be that much more congruent. This, again, has implications for counselling. The thing that causes many people discomfort in their lives is, arguably, that they have a particular view or set of beliefs about the world that does not match reality. This, in turn, may lead to the sort of thinking that is prefaced by expressions such as 'if only . . .', 'things would be much easier if . . .', 'I know there's no point in thinking like this, but . . .'. All such thoughts tend to lead to a distorted picture of what is actually happening in a person's life. Part of the process of counselling may be to enable people to identify these false perceptions and to clarify them. This is not to argue that there is one sure way of looking at the world but that people need to be happy that what goes on in their heads bears a reasonable resemblance to how things actually are in the world.

So, too, must the counsellor work at the process of clarifying her thoughts in line with what she actually perceives about the world. This can be done in a variety of ways: through talking things through with a colleague or a friend, through reading and continuing education and through introspection – the process of looking inward and exploring what the poet Gerard Manley Hopkins called the 'inscape' (Hopkins, 1953).

Feelings

Feeling refers to the emotional aspect of the person: joy, love, anger, disappointment and so forth. Heron (1977a) argues that in our present society we have learned to repress many of our feelings because the cultural norm dictates that we do not overtly express them, particularly the stronger expressions of anger, tears, fear and embarrassment. He argues, also, that such repression leads to the person carrying with them a great deal of unexpressed feeling that acts as a block to rational thinking, creativity and general enjoyment of life.

Counselling is frequently concerned with allowing people to express such pent-up emotions and there seems to be a direct link between the degree to which a counsellor can freely and appropriately express her own emotions and the degree to which she can allow the client to express his. It seems that if we block a lot of our own stronger feelings, when we are faced with another person who wants to express feelings, we feel reticent about allowing them to do so. Very often, this is because the other person's emotion stirs up memories of our own feelings. As we have hung on to them for so long, a mechanism seems to come into play that encourages us to disallow that expression in others and thus allows us to carry on holding on to our own.

A simple experiment may demonstrate the degree to which we carry around bottled-up emotion. Next time you feel moved to tears by something that you see on television, switch off the set and allow yourself to cry. Then listen inwardly to what you are crying about. The chances are that it will be something to do with your own personal history rather than being related directly to what you saw on the screen.

The health professional who counsels people who wish to express pent-up feelings should seriously consider exploring their own emotional status. This can be done through the medium of counselling supervision, in which the counsellor meets regularly with another trained counsellor and talks through and explores their work load. It can also be achieved through the process known as co-counselling, which is described in Chapter 9. It can also help to join a peer support group (Ernst and Goodison, 1981) in which feelings can be explored in a safe and supportive atmosphere. Such support groups can be instituted and facilitated by a number of like-thinking colleagues and can do much to relieve the pressure of working with the emotionally stressed. Without such support, the health professional can easily slip into a position where she can no longer help the person who wants to express feelings because her own emotional needs are not catered for. The net result, as we noted earlier, can be burnout – a feeling of profound physical and emotional exhaustion caused by job-related stress. Self-awareness, then, involves not only the thinking side of the person but also the feeling or emotional side.

Sensing

Sensing refers to inputs through the five special senses: touch, taste, smell, hearing, sight and also to proprioceptive and kinaesthetic sense. Proprioception refers to our ability to know the position of our bodies and thus to know where we are in space. We may note, for instance, that we do not have to think whether or not we are sitting down or standing up: we know that through our proprioceptive sense, through bundles of nerve fibres which constantly feed the information back to our brains. Kinaesthetic sense refers to our sense of body movement. Again, this is a sense that we do not normally have to think about – we just move!

Much of the time, we are not aware of the potential stimulation that exists for our senses: we filter out many of the stimuli. A short experiment will illustrate how this filtering process works. Stop reading this book for a moment and pay attention to everything coming in through your senses. What can you hear? What can you see? What can you smell? What can you taste? What can you feel? In recognizing these various inputs through the senses, it becomes apparent just how much is normally not noticed in the course of a day. Now, for much of the time, such filtering out is useful in that it allows us to concentrate on a particular task in hand. In terms of counselling, however, it is vital that we learn to develop an acute awareness of the inputs coming in through the senses, particularly those of hearing and of sight. When counselling, we are not only hearing what the client is saying but also paying attention to how they say it – their tone of voice, the inflection, the volume of their voice and so on. Further, we need to pay attention to the client's appearance in terms of how they are dressed, how they sit and how they use non-verbal communication: eye contact, body movement, touch, proximity to the counsellor and so forth. Without an awareness of these points of communication, we lose a lot of important information that can guide us in deciding how best to intervene in the counselling relationship.

Fortunately, the process of developing such awareness is, in one sense, easy – we just have to do it! If time is set aside each day just to notice what is going on around us, we can quickly learn to extend this period until we are much more acutely aware of sensory input. Such noticing can become a way of life. The process of noticing is often blocked, however, by internal distraction – recurrent thoughts and worries. Clearly, it is less easy to pay such close attention to what is going on around us when our lives are particularly stressful and we are preoccupied for much of the time with some sort of 'internal dialogue'. Certainly, we cannot be effective counsellors unless we can give almost total attention to the client and therefore, at times of personal emotional stress, the health professional is likely to function less well in the capacity of counsellor. This, perhaps, is another reason why the person regularly acting in a counselling role should seriously consider peer support of some sort. Such support is not only useful in talking through difficult issues in counselling, but it may also help the counsellor to work through some of their own problems in living.

Intuiting

The intuitive aspect of the person is perhaps the most undervalued. Intuiting refers to knowledge and insight that arrives independently of the senses. Ornstein (1975), in a study of the two sides of the brain, came to the conclusion that the intuitive function is associated with the right side of the brain, whilst the more cognitive process is associated with the left. If Ornstein is right, the implication is that if the intuitive aspect is developed further, then both sides of the brain will function optimally. Certainly, Ornstein sees the two processes as complementary and argues, with Jung, that the intuitive side of the person should be developed alongside the more cognitive aspect. Western culture tends to be dominated by the left brain approach to education and development; certainly, rationality is usually viewed as more important than intuition. Ornstein places intuition beyond mere intellectual understanding in terms of importance and suggests the use of metaphors, allegories, music and Sufi fables as the means by which intuition can be developed.

It may be the case that the intuitive aspect of the person is neglected through fear that it may not be trusted. It is probably true that most of us have intended to act at some time from an intuitive feeling but have held back at the last minute because we could not be sure that our intuition was right. On the other hand, many aspects of the counselling process demand an intuitive approach. In order to empathize with another person, we are required to grasp intuitively what it is to be like them. Certainly, very sensitive issues require an intuitive approach – mere logic or rationality is somehow not enough. Carl Rogers (1967) noted that whenever he felt a hunch about something that was happening in the counselling relationship, it invariably helped if he verbalized it, although he acknowledged, too, that he often also doubted his own intuitive ability and took the rational approach, only to find out later that his hunch had been accurate! Using intuition consciously and openly takes courage but used alongside more rational approaches, it can enhance the counselling relationship in a way that logic never can.

On the other hand, once again it is necessary to note that intuition is an abstraction – it does not have concrete reality that we can point to. Some of the situations in which we posit intuition as having played a part may be explained in other ways. For example, sometimes I think I have discovered something 'intuitively' simply because I have forgotten that I had learned the fact before. Sometimes, I may anticipate what someone else will say 'intuitively' because I have got to know them quite well and know the sorts of things that this person *does* say. Not everything we think of as 'intuitive' may be so. Of course, there are still plenty of things that happen that we cannot give a better name to than 'intuition'.

These four internal aspects of the person – thinking, feeling, sensing and intuiting – need to be developed in combination. Jung argued that many people rely heavily on a one-sided approach, particularly the thinking/sensing approach. Such people, he argued, prefer rational argument, backed up by evidence through the senses of a fairly concrete nature. In other words, such people dismiss what they cannot directly see, hear, taste, smell or touch or which cannot be rationally argued about. Such a position, whilst clearly safe, arguably discounts some of the more subtle and even metaphysical aspects of life. Certainly it tends to denigrate emotional experience and, presumably, dismisses intuition on the grounds of its not being rational! In terms of the counselling relationship, it would seem valuable to develop all four aspects of the self for it is those four aspects that the client very often has problems with. Life problems are not always of the rational, thinking sort. Nor are they concerned only with what can be directly sensed. Many problems in living are directly related to emotions, feelings and sometimes 'un-nameable' problems – problems concerned with the intuitive domain. Herman Hesse (1979) sums up the problems of these sorts of issues, our tendency to ignore the feeling and intuitive domains and our temptation to seek, too readily, clarification through rationality.

> ***. . . each of us paints and misrepresents every day and every hour the jungle of mysteries, transforming it into a pretty garden or a flat, neatly drawn map, the moralist with the help of his maxims, the man of religion with the help of his faith, the engineer with the help of his slide-rule, the painter with the help of his palette, and the poet with the help of his examples and ideals. And each one of us lives completely and content and assured in his pseudo-world and on his map, just so long as he does not feel, through some breach in the dam or some frightful flash of lightning, reality, the monster, the terrifying beauty, the appalling horror, falling upon him, inescapably embracing him and lethally taking him prisoner.***

The experience of the body

Another aspect of this integrated model of the self is the experience of the body. If, as has been argued, the mind and body are inextricably linked, then any mental activity will manifest itself as some sort of bodily change and vice versa. It is notable, however, how often we divide the two up. Expressions such as 'my mind is OK, it's my body that's the problem' and 'I'm not happy with my body' indicate how easy it is to make this distinction. A moment's reflection, however, will reveal how artificial this distinction really is. In fact, we do not *have* a mind and a body, we are our mind and body. When we speak of the self, we are speaking of both aspects – mind and body.

Coming to notice the sometimes small changes that take place in the mind/body takes time and patience. Stop reading for a moment and consider your own body. What do you notice? Do you have areas of muscle tension – in the shoulders or neck, for example? What parts of the body are you not aware of? Have any bodily sensations changed since you started noticing? What is your breathing like? Fast, slow, deep or shallow? Many of these small changes in the body tempo can help us to locate changes in mood. Often the first symptom of a mood or state of mind is a bodily change. In learning to notice the body, we can learn to make valuable observations about ourselves and thus further develop self-awareness. Such noticing is also of value in the counselling relationship, for a client's emotions are also often expressed in physical terms. A sudden change of breathing rate can indicate rising anxiety, for example. Psychological tension is often expressed in the form of tightened muscles.

Learning to listen to the body in this way can help us more accurately to assess our true feelings about ourselves and others. Wilhelm Reich (1949), a contemporary of Freud and a psychoanalyst who was particularly interested in the mind–body relationship, argued that many of us carry around with us unexpressed emotion that is somehow 'stored' in our musculature. Emotions, then, could become trapped in sets of muscles. He maintained that direct manipulation of those muscles could release the emotion trapped within them. Such therapy applied directly to the body has become known as Reichian bodywork and can be a powerful means of releasing pent-up emotion and gaining self-awareness through a very direct method.

Similar but different versions of this physical approach to psychological issues may be found in bioenergetics (Lowen, 1967), Feldenkrais (Feldenkrais, 1972) and the Alexander technique (Alexander, 1969). Other examples of the approach to self-awareness through the mind/body include massage, yoga, the martial arts, certain types of meditation, dance and certain sorts of sports and exercise.

All these methods can enhance self-awareness through attention to changes in the body and thus create insight into psychological states. They can also aid development of awareness of body image. If we notice people in everyday life, we may observe how many people walk in a lopsided manner or stoop their shoulders and may even have different sorts of expressions on either side of their face! Bodywork methods may help in balancing the person and may lead to a greater sense of physical (and, therefore, psychological) symmetry. It would seem reasonable to argue that it would be strange to concentrate on developing awareness of the mind whilst totally ignoring the body. Similarly, it is perhaps odd to concentrate on physical fitness or balance without paying attention to psychological status. This joint focus also applies to the process of counselling. Effective counselling involves paying attention to both what the client says and what he does. Thus the mind/body is attended to as a totality.

This, then, is an integrated model of the self, focusing on the outer, public expression of self through our behaviour and an inner, more private aspect of self. Clearly, this is only one way of discussing the self and as we noted earlier, the self has many facets, including the self-as-perceived-by-others. The model offered here, however, may allow us to start developing self-awareness as an important tool in the process of skilful counselling. For self-awareness can never be developed purely for its own sake, but as a means of enhancing our caring and helping skills.

SELF-AWARENESS

What is self-awareness? First, the point needs to be made that it is not self-consciousness in the sense of becoming painfully aware of how we imagine other people see us. Sartre (1956) describes this condition well saying that when we come under the scrutinizing gaze of another person, we perceive ourselves as being turned into objects by that other person. It is as though we become a thing rather than a person. Such a notion of treating people as things and the resultant self-consciousness is a valuable concept in the context of counselling, for it is important that we do not concentrate on the *problems* of the person we are counselling to the extent that they merely become interesting cases. Once we do this, we have made them into things and as a result they may feel distinctly uncared for and uncomfortable.

Self-awareness is the evolving and expanding sense of noticing and taking account of a wide range of aspects of self. As we explore our psychological and physical make-up we get to know ourselves better. Chapman and Gale (1982) note a curious paradox about this process, in that gaining knowledge of something does not normally change that thing. If, for instance, I learn an equation, that equation does not change as a result of my having learnt it. With self-awareness, however, the subject of the learning – the self – changes as more is learnt about it. In this sense, then, the process of developing self-awareness is a continuous process because we are continuously changing. Self-awareness, curiously, may speed up that change.

Two different and complementary methods of developing self-awareness may be described. One is through the process of introspection or looking inward. The other is through receiving feedback about ourselves from other people. The two used in balance can lead to a reasonable and hopefully accurate picture of the self. One without the other can lead to a curiously skewed sense of self. Thus, introspection on its own can lead to either an unnecessarily harsh judgement of the self or a narcissistic and self-centred view. Relying only on feedback from others can lead us to concentrate only on the external or public aspect of the self. Again, there is no guarantee that another person's assessment of us is any more or less accurate than our own but it is important to hear it! To be able to hear it undefensively is yet another skill. Often, when other people tell us what they think of us, for good or bad, we react to it. The skill here may be to

Aspects of self-awareness	Methods of developing self-awareness
1. *Thinking, including:* – stream of consciousness – belief systems – ideas – fantasies etc	Discussion/conversation Group work Introspection Brainstorming Meditation Writing Use of problem-solving cycle, etc.
2. *Feelings including:* – anger – fear – grief – embarrassment – joy/happiness – mood swings etc.	Discussion/conversation Group work Introspection Gestalt exercises Meditation Co-counselling Supervision Analysis Cathartic work Sensitivity training Encounter group work Role play, etc.
3. *Sensations, including:* – taste – touch – hearing – smell – sight etc.	Focussing attention on one or more sensations at a time Group exercises Use of sensory stimulation/deprivation exercises, gestalt exercises Noticing in everyday life, etc.
4. *Sexuality, including:* – orientation (heterosexual/homosexual/bisexual) – expression of sexuality etc.	Discussion/conversation Counselling/co-counselling Values, clarification exercises, etc.
5. *Spirituality, including:* – belief systems – life philosophy – awareness of choice – varieties of religious experience – atheism and agnosticism etc.	Discussion/conversation Group work Meditation Prayer Reading Aesthetic experience (art, music, poetry, etc.) Life planning, goal setting

continued

Figure 3.2

Methods of developing self-awareness.

accept it, in much the same way as it has been suggested that we accept what the client says to us in counselling. If we can free others to tell us easily their impression of us, we are slightly more likely to get an honest view from them on other occasions. This has implications for work in peer support groups used as vehicles for self-awareness development. Just as we must be prepared to listen fully to the client in counselling, so we must be prepared to listen fully to our peers in such a group.

Aspects of self-awareness	Methods of developing self-awareness
6. *Physical status, including:* – the body systems – health status etc	 Self-examination Medical examination Exercise Sport Martial arts Meditation Massage Bodywork, etc.
7. *Appearance, including:* – dress – personal style – height, weight etc.	 Discussion/conversation Self- and peer assessment Self-monitoring Use of video, etc.
8. *Knowledge, including:* – level of propositional knowledge – level of practical knowledge – level of experiential knowledge	 Discussion/conversation Group work Examinations/testing/quizzing Study Use of distance-learning packages Enrolment on courses Self- and peer assessment etc.
9. *Needs and wants, including:* – financial/material – physical – love and belonging – achievement – knowledge – aesthetic – spiritual – self-actualization etc.	 Discussion/conversation Group work Values clarification work Assertiveness training Lifestyle evaluation etc.
10. *Spirituality, including:* – verbal and non-verbal skills – values – unknown/undiscovered aspects of the self	 Discussion/conversation Counselling/co-counselling Self-analysis Social skills training

Figure 3.2

Methods of developing self-awareness, continued.

Figure 3.2 offers a variety of practical methods for developing self-awareness that may be used by the individual working on her own or by groups of peers working together in a group. It is not suggested that it represents an exhaustive list of self-awareness methods, but it can serve as a starting point. In practice, the individual will often identify particular preferences for certain methods of self-awareness development. It is important, however, to occasionally 'freshen the act' and try new methods!

It is important to note that self-awareness development should be an enjoyable process. It should neither be too earnest nor too concentrated. A sense of perspective and a sense of humour are essential to the process as is keeping a sense of the 'larger picture' – the social situation in which the individual exists. A political and social awareness is vital to the development of counselling skills as is a sense of self-awareness.

SELF-AWARENESS AND THE HEALTH PROFESSIONAL

As we have seen, self-awareness underlies almost every aspect of the counselling relationship. In all the health professions, the fact that the professional forms close and personal relationships with her clients emphasizes this need for understanding of the self. When other people are physically, emotionally, socially or spiritually distressed, that distress cannot but affect us too. We need not only professional knowledge and know-how, related to our particular speciality and an awareness of how our work fits in with the work of others in the caring team, but also personal awareness that can inform our practice in the health field. Such self-awareness can help us to develop an understanding of the basic principles of counselling discussed in the next chapter.

4 Basic principles and considerations

In order to function effectively as a counsellor, it is necessary to consider some principles that can enhance or detract from the relationship. First, we shall look at what may be considered the ideal counselling relationship. Fiedler, in 1950, asked a wide variety of counsellors what they considered to be the ingredients of an ideal therapeutic relationship. The list that was generated by his research included the following:

1 an empathic relationship;
2 the therapist and patient relate well;
3 the therapist sticks closely to the patient's problems;
4 the patient feels free to say what he likes;
5 an atmosphere of mutual trust and confidence exists;
6 rapport is excellent.

Note, again, that many of these points are abstractions. What, for example, does it mean to 'relate well' and what does it mean to say that 'rapport is excellent' and who decides?

In 1957, Carl Rogers developed Fiedler's work and identified what he called the six necessary and sufficient conditions for therapeutic change via the counselling relationship. He argued that the following conditions had to exist and continue for a period if counselling was to be effective.

1 Two persons are in psychological contact.
2 The first, whom we shall term the client, is in a state of incongruence – vulnerable or anxious.
3 The second person, whom we shall term the therapist, is congruent or integrated in the relationship.
4 The therapist experiences unconditional regard for the client.
5 The therapist experiences an empathic understanding of the client's internal frame of reference and endeavours to communicate this experience to the client.
6 The communication to the client of the therapist's empathic understanding and unconditional positive regard is to a minimal degree achieved.

There are various problems that we may identify with Roger's list. First, it is not clear what it means to be 'in psychological contact'. Second, we cannot assume, perhaps, that all clients are necessarily 'incongruent' (and, indeed, it is possible to question what this might mean). Third, we might question what it is meant by the therapist becoming 'congruent and integrated in the relationship'.

Whether or not Rogers' claim of these conditions being necessary and sufficient is completely accurate in the philosophical sense of those terms need not concern us here. What is particularly useful is that the list identifies certain personal qualities that must exist in the person in order for them to function as an effective counsellor. The particular personal qualities that Rogers discusses frequently in his writing about counselling are unconditional positive regard, empathic understanding, warmth and genuineness (Rogers, 1967). The need for these qualities is also borne out by the research conducted by Truax and Carkuff (1967) and the characteristics of empathy, warmth and genuineness are often referred to as the 'Truax triad' (Schulman, 1982). To these qualities may be added those of concreteness and immediacy, also suggested by Carkuff (1969). All these qualities are worth exploring further as they can lay the foundations for effective counselling in any context.

NECESSARY PERSONAL QUALITIES OF THE EFFECTIVE COUNSELLOR

Unconditional positive regard

Rogers' rather clumsy phrase conveys a particularly important predisposition towards the client, by the counsellor. It is also called *prizing* or even just *accepting*. It means that the client is viewed with dignity and valued as a worthwhile and positive human being. The 'unconditional' prefix refers to the idea that such regard is offered without any preconditions. Often in relationships, some sort of reciprocity is demanded: I will like you (or love you) as long as you return that liking or loving. Rogers is asking that the feelings that the counsellor holds for the client should be undemanding and not require reciprocation. Also, there is a suggestion of an inherent goodness within the client. This notion of persons as essentially good can be traced back, at least to Rousseau's *Emile* and is possibly philosophically problematic. Notions such as goodness and badness are social constructions and to argue that a person is born good or bad is fraught with difficulties. However, as a practical starting point in the counselling relationship, it seems to be a good idea that we assume an inherent, positive and life-asserting characteristic in the client. It seems difficult to argue otherwise. It would be odd, for instance, to engage in the process of counselling with the view that the person was essentially bad, negative and unlikely to grow or develop! Thus, unconditional positive regard offers a baseline from which to start the counselling relationship. In order to further grasp this concept, it may be useful to refer directly to Rogers' definition of the notion.

> *I hypothesize that growth and change are more likely to occur the more that the counsellor is experiencing a warm, positive, acceptant attitude towards what is the client. It means that he prizes the client, as a person, with the same quality of feeling that a parent feels for his child, prizing him as a person regardless of his particular behaviour at the moment. It means that he cares for his client in a non-possessive way, as a person with potentialities. It involves an open willingness for the*

> *client to be whatever feelings are real in him at the moment – hostility or tenderness, rebellion or submissiveness, assurance or self-depreciation. It means a kind of love for the client as he is, providing we understand the word love as equivalent to the theologian's term agape and not in its usual romantic and possessive meanings. What I am describing is a feeling which is not paternalistic, nor sentimental, nor superficially social and agreeable. It respects the other person as a separate individual and does not possess him. It is a kind of liking which has strength, and which is not demanding. We have termed it positive regard. (Rogers and Stevens, 1967)*

Unconditional positive regard, then, involves a deep and positive feeling for the other person, perhaps equivalent in the health professions to what Alistair Campbell has called 'moderated love' (Campbell, 1984). He talks of 'lovers and professors,' suggesting that certain professionals profess to love, thus claiming both the ability to be professional and to express altruistic love or disinterested love for others. The suggestion is also that the health professional has a positive and warm confidence in her own skills and abilities in the counselling relationship. Halmos (1965) sums this up when he writes:

> *'You are worthwhile!' and 'I am not put off by your illness!' This moral stance of not admitting defeat is possible for those who have faith or a kind of stubborn confidence in the rightness of what they are doing.*

For Halmos, the counselling relationship is something of an act of faith. There can be no guarantee that the counselling offered will be effective but the counsellor enters the relationship with the belief that it will be. It is this positive outlook in the counsellor and this positive belief in the ability of the client to change for the better that is summarized in Rogers' notion of unconditional positive regard (Rogers and Stevens, 1967). Such an outlook is also supported by Egan (1982) who, in his 'portrait of a helper', says:

> *They respect their clients and express this respect by being available to them, working with them, not judging them, trusting the constructive forces found in them, and ultimately placing the expectation on them that they will do whatever is necessary to handle their problems in living more effectively.*

Empathic understanding

Empathy is the ability to enter the perceptual world of the other person: to see the world as they see it. It also suggests an ability to convey this identification of feelings to the other person. Kalisch (1971) defines empathy as 'the ability to perceive accurately the feelings of another person and to communicate this understanding to him' whilst Mayeroff (1972), in a classic book on caring, describes empathic understanding from this point of view of caring for another person.

> *To care for another person I must be able to understand him and his world as if I were inside it. I must be able to see, as it were, with his eyes what his world is like to him and how he sees himself. Instead of merely looking at him in a detached way from outside, as if he were a specimen, I must be able to be with him in his world, 'going' into his world in order to sense from 'inside' what life is like for him, what he is striving to be, and what he requires to grow.*

Empathy is clearly different from sympathy. Sympathy suggests feeling sorry for the other person or, perhaps, identifying with how they feel. If I sympathize, I imagine myself as being in the other person's position and how I would feel. If I empathize, however, I try to imagine how it is to be the other person – feeling sorry for him does not really come into the issue.

As with unconditional positive regard, the process of developing empathy involves something of an act of faith. When we empathize with another person, we cannot know what the outcome will be. If we pre-empt the outcome of our empathizing, we are already not empathizing – we are thinking of solutions and ways of influencing the client towards a particular goal that we have in mind. The process of empathizing involves entering into the perceptual world of the other person without necessarily knowing where that process will lead to. Martin Buber, the Hassidic philosopher, mystic and writer on psychotherapy, summed up well this mixture of willingness to explore the world of the other without presupposing the outcome when he wrote:

> *A man lost his way in a great forest. After a while another lost his way and chanced on the first. Without knowing what had happened to him, he asked the way out of the woods. 'I don't know,' said the first. 'But I can point out the ways that lead further into the thicket, and after that let us try to find the way together.' (Buber, 1948)*

The process of developing empathic understanding is the process of exploring the client's world with the client, neither judging nor suggesting. It can be achieved best through the process of careful attending and listening to the other person and, perhaps, by use of the skill known as *reflection*, discussed in a later chapter (p. 125). Essentially, though, it is also a way of being, a disposition towards the client, a willingness to explore and intuitively allow the other person to express themselves fully. Again, as with unconditional positive regard and with all aspects of the client-centred approach to counselling, the empathic approach is underpinned by the idea that it is the client in the end who will find his own way through and will find his own, idiosyncratic answers to his problems in living. To be empathic is to be a fellow traveller, a friend to the person as they undertake the search. Empathic understanding, then, involves the notion of befriending alluded to in Chapter 1. Just as a friend can (usually!) accept another friend 'warts and all', so the counsellor, in being empathic, is offering such acceptance.

There are, of course, limitations to the degree to which we can truly empathize. Because we all live in different worlds based on our particular culture, education, physiology, belief systems and so forth, we all view that world slightly differently. Thus, truly empathizing with another person would involve actually becoming that other person! Clearly impossible! We can, however, strive to get as close to the perceptual world of the other by listening and attending and by suspending judgement. We can also learn to forget ourselves temporarily and give ourselves as completely as we can to the other person.

In the following dialogue, a young girl, Rebecca, is talking to her social worker, about the situation at home. The dialogue illustrates something of the nature of developing empathy.

Rebecca: I don't know, I just don't seem to be getting on with people.
Social worker: When you say people?
Rebecca: I mean my parents. They don't have any idea.
Social worker: They don't have any idea about you?
Rebecca: No, they think that I want to stay at school and go to university and everything. Well, I do, in a way. But I wish they wouldn't push me all the time! They think they have to tell me how to do things all the time.
Social worker: It's as if they want to push you in a certain direction and you're not sure whether or not you want to go that way.
Rebecca: That's exactly it! I don't know what I want to do any more! They push me so much that I don't know what I want!
Social worker: And that's upsetting you?
Rebecca: Yeah, a lot . . . I get upset easily these days and I'm sure it's got a lot to do with what's happening at home.

In this example, the two people become closely involved in the conversation and the social worker, rather than directing the conversation in a particular way, follows the thoughts and feelings that Rebecca expresses. Empathy is developed through this following process and through a willingness to listen to both what is said and what is implied. An intuitive ability is just as important in empathy as is technical skill.

Barrett-Lennard (1981, 1993) writes of the *empathy cycle model* and viewed empathy as an intentional, purposeful activity, developed by the counsellor. He envisaged the empathy cycle as comprising five stages, as follows.

Stage 1: empathic set of the counsellor. The client is actively expressing some aspect of his or her experiencing. The counsellor is actively attending and receptive.
Stage 2: empathic resonation. The counsellor resonates to the directly or indirectly expressed aspects of the client's experiencing.
Stage 3: expressed empathy. The counsellor expresses or communicates his or her felt awareness of the client's experiencing.

Stage 4: received empathy. The client is attending to the counsellor sufficiently to form a sense of perception of the counsellor's immediate personal understanding.

Stage 5: the empathy cycle continues. The client then continues or resumes self-expression in a way that provides feedback to the counsellor concerning the accuracy of the empathic response and the quality of the therapeutic relationship. (Barrett-Lennard, 1981)

Although Barrett-Lennard's representation of empathy is a little wordy, this cycle highlights the *process* aspect of empathy and the need not only for the counsellor to express empathy but also for the client to be able to *experience* it.

Warmth and genuineness

Warmth in the counselling relationship refers to a certain approachability and willingness to be open with the client. Schulman (1982) notes that the following characteristics are included in the concept of warmth: equal worth, absence of blame, non-defensiveness and closeness. Warmth is a frame of mind rather than a skill and perhaps one developed through being honest with oneself and being prepared to be open with others. It is also about treating the other person as an equal human being. Martin Buber (1958) distinguishes between the I–it relationship and the I–thou (or I–you) relationship. In the I–it relationship, one person treats the other as an object, a thing. In the I–thou relationship, there occurs a meeting of persons, despite any differences there may be in terms of status, background, lifestyle, belief or value systems. In the I–thou relationship there is a sense of mutuality, a sense that can be contagious and is of particular value in the counselling relationship.

> *In a meaningful friendship, caring is mutual, each cares for the other; caring becomes contagious. My caring for the other helps activate his caring for me; and similarly his caring for me helps activate my caring for him, it 'strengthens' me to care for him. (Mayeroff, 1972)*

What is less clear, however, is the degree to which a counselling relationship can be a mutual relationship. Rogers (1967) argues that the counselling relationship can be a mutual relationship but Buber acknowledges that because it is always the client who seeks out the counsellor and comes to that counsellor with problems, the relationship is necessarily unequal and lacking in mutuality.

> *He comes for help to you. You don't come for help to him. And not only this, but you are able, more or less, to help him. He can do different things to you, but not help you . . . You are, of course, a very important person for him. But not a person whom he wants to see and to know and is able to. He is floundering around, he comes to you. He is, may I say, entangled in your life, in your thoughts, in your being, your*

> ***communication, and so on. But he is not interested in you as you. It cannot be. (Buber, 1966)***

Thus warmth must be offered by the counsellor but the feeling will not necessarily be reciprocated by the client. There is another problem with the notion of warmth. We each perceive personal qualities in different sorts of ways. One person's warmth is another person's patronage or sentimentality. We cannot guarantee how our presentation of self will be perceived by the other person. In a more general way, however, warmth may be compared to coldness. It is clear that the cold person would not be the ideal person to undertake counselling! Further, our relationships with others tend to be self-monitoring to a degree: we anticipate, as we go, the effect we are having on others and modify our presentation of self accordingly. Thus, we soon get to know if our warmth is suffocating the client or is being perceived by him in a negative way. This ability to constantly monitor ourselves and our relationships is an important part of the process of developing counselling skills.

Genuineness, too, is an important facet of the relationship. We either care for the person in front of us or we do not. We cannot fake professional interest. We must be interested. Clearly, some people will interest us more than others. Often, those clients who remind us at some level of our own problems or our own personalities will interest us most of all. This is not so important as our having a genuine interest in the fact that the relationship is happening at all. The strength of interest is not the important issue but the commitment to involvement is.

There may appear to be a conflict between the concept of genuineness and the self-monitoring alluded to above. Self-monitoring may be viewed as artificial or contrived and therefore not genuine. The genuineness discussed here relates to the counsellor's interest in the human relationship that is developing between the two people. Any ways in which that relationship can be enhanced must serve a valuable purpose. It is quite possible to be genuine and yet aware of what is happening: genuine and yet committed to increasing interpersonal competence.

Genuineness starts with self-awareness. This is summed up in Shakespeare's observation:

> *This above all – to thine own self be true;*
> *And it must follow, as the night the day,*
> *Thou canst not then be false to any man. (Hamlet, Act 1, Scene 3)*

Egan (1990) sums up the notion of genuineness in the context of counselling when he identifies the following aspects of it.

> *You are genuine in your relationship with your clients when you:*
>
> - *do not overemphasize your professional role and avoid stereotyped role behaviours;*

- ***are spontaneous but not uncontrolled or haphazard in your relationships;***
- ***remain open and non-defensive even when you feel threatened;***
- ***are consistent and avoid discrepancies – between your values and your behaviour, and between your thoughts and your words in interactions with clients – while remaining respectful and reasonably tactful;***
- ***are willing to share yourself and your experience with clients if it seems helpful.***

> ***Reflecting on counselling***
>
> The discussion about personal qualities of the counsellor hinges on the idea that we are all in agreement about what constitutes 'warmth', 'empathy' and so on. Is this assumption sound? It might be argued that one person's 'warmth' is another person's 'sickliness'. It is worth considering to what degree there is general agreement about the use of these terms.

Concreteness

Concreteness refers to the idea that the counsellor should be clear and explicit in her dealings with the client and should help the client to express himself clearly. This is essential if communication between the two parties is to be successful. Concreteness involves helping the client to put into words those things that are only being hinted at in order that both client and counsellor understand what the client is perceiving at any given time. The following conversation demonstrates the counsellor attempting to develop this sense of concreteness.

Client: I don't know, I feel sort of disinterested a lot of the time . . . as if no-one cared much about what was going on.
Counsellor: You seem to be saying two things: you feel disinterested and you feel that no-one cares for you.
Client: They're not interested in what I do.
Counsellor: Other people aren't interested in you?
Client: Yes, that's right. I'm OK . . . it's just that other people don't want to know about me.
Counsellor: When you say other people, who do you mean?
Client: You know . . . my family . . . my wife especially.

In this way, the counsellor helps the client to clarify what he is saying and enables him to be more specific. Without such clarification it is possible for both parties to be talking to each other without either really understanding the other. Whenever the counsellor senses that she is losing the client it is useful for her to return to this concrete approach.

It is important, too, that the counsellor does not mystify the client by overpowering him with technique or with unasked-for interpretations. This is another sense of the notion of being concrete. The client should at no time feel threatened by the counselling relationship nor feel that the counsellor is 'doing something strange'. Sometimes, the person new to counselling will feel more comfortable hiding behind a mystique and a sense of being a therapist. Such behaviour cuts across the notions of remaining warm and empathic. The counselling relationship should remain clear and unmysterious to the client. Rogers (1967) has used the word *transparent* to describe this sense of openness and clarity.

Immediacy

When people are distressed by the life situation in which they find themselves, there is a temptation for them to spend a considerable amount of time reminiscing about the past. Somehow, it seems safer to talk of the past rather than face feelings in the here-and-now. One of the tasks of the counsellor is to help the client to identify present thoughts and feelings. In this way, current issues are addressed and problem solving can relate directly to those present-day issues. This is not to say that the client should never be allowed to talk about the past but to note that the counsellor may function more effectively if they keep a check on the degree to which such reminiscing occurs. In a sense, the present is all there is: the past is past and the future has not yet arrived. The client who talks excessively about how things were avoids the reality of the present.

'DON'TS' IN THE COUNSELLING RELATIONSHIP

Having identified some of the qualities and characteristics of an effective counselling relationship, it is time to turn to some things that do not enhance it. These can be discussed most easily in the form of a list of 'don'ts'. Like any such list, there will be occasions on which any one of these items may be helpful in the counselling relationship: that is an illustration of how such relationships are unique and unpredictable! As a general rule, however, the following issues run contrary to the qualities identified above and are best avoided.

Don't ask 'why' questions

(Example: Why do you feel depressed?)

The word 'why' suggests interrogation, probing and a sense of disapproval. Further, the 'why' question can encourage the client to discuss their feelings in a theoretical way. In other words, when the counsellor asks the client why he is depressed, she is inviting him to offer a theory about why he feels that way. In the following example of dialogue between a community psychiatric nurse and her patient, we see this shift from feelings to theory.

Nurse: Tell me a bit more about how you're feeling at the moment.
Patient: It's difficult to say . . . I feel depressed, really.

Nurse: Why do you feel like that?
Patient: My mother was depressive . . . perhaps I take after her . . .

The 'why' question in this example does nothing to help the patient expand on his expression of feeling but leads him immediately to offer a theoretical explanation of his feelings. 'Why' questions are best avoided altogether in the context of counselling, although a considerable effort may have to be exerted on the part of the new counsellor to drop them from her repertoire! 'Why' questions tend to be very frequent in everyday conversation and the temptation to ask them can be very strong. Perhaps, too, they derive from an almost inherent sense of nosiness that most of us feel at some time or another!

Don't use 'shoulds' and 'oughts'

(Example: You realize that what you should do is . . .)

Moralizing rarely helps. When the counsellor suggests what the other person should do, she forces her own frame of reference, her own value system, on the client. It is difficult to imagine many situations in which a counsellor can really advise another person about what they should do. Possible exceptions to this rule are those situations in which concrete facts are under discussion. For example, a doctor may suggest that a patient should finish a course of medicine. In counselling, however, the issues under discussion are usually the client's problems in living. The counsellor's value system is rarely of use in helping the client to untangle his life and find a solution to his problem.

Don't blame

(Example: I'm not surprised, you've been very stupid.)

As with the question of 'oughts' and 'shoulds', trying to suggest or apportion blame is not constructive. In a sense, it doesn't matter who is to blame in any particular situation. The point is that a situation has occurred and the client is trying to find ways of dealing with it.

Don't automatically compare the client's experience with your own experience

(Example: I know exactly what you mean . . . I'm like that too . . .)

The key word here is 'automatically'. Sometimes, shared experience can be helpful to the client. Often, however, it can lead to an exchange of experiences that is neither helpful nor progressive. Luft (1969) uses the descriptor *parallaction* to describe the sorts of parallel conversations that can occur as a result of such comparison. In the following example, two friends are discussing the previous evening.

I had a good night, last night. Went to the cinema.
Yes, we went out to a restaurant.
I hadn't seen a film for months.
We don't get out for meals very often.

I saw *Gone With the Wind* . . . it must be 30 years old!
Have you seen David in the last few weeks?

In the conversation, neither person is really listening to the other. Each wants to talk about himself and neither is prepared to hear the other. Clearly, such an exaggerated situation is unlikely to occur in counselling, but it is surprising how such comparisons of experience can lead down blind alleys. An example of how this can occur is as follows. The conversation is between a social worker and her client.

Client: I get very anxious, sometimes . . . especially when I've got exams coming up.
Social worker: I suppose everybody does . . . I know I do . . .
Client: I get to think that I won't make it . . . that I'm not good enough.
Social worker: I know what you mean. I thought I wouldn't get my social work exams . . . I got really upset.

The counselling relationship belongs to the client: it is his time to explore his problems. If the counsellor constantly compares her own experience with that of the client, she is taking away some of that time from the client. More importantly, perhaps, she is saying to the client, 'Your problems are my problems'. And yet, it is the client who is coming to see the counsellor and not vice versa! It is likely that if the counsellor expresses such similarity of experience to the client, the latter will resent it for how can it be that both have similar problems and yet one has to approach the other for help in solving those problems? Such a contradiction can confuse and irritate the client and spoil the counselling relationship.

Don't invalidate the client's feelings

(Example: Of course you're not angry/depressed/in love . . . you just think you are . . .)

This sort of judgement is a curious one. It suggests a number of possibilities: (a) the client is not telling the truth; (b) the client doesn't use words appropriately (presumably in accordance with the counsellor's definitions!); or (c) the counsellor is better able to judge the client's feelings than the client himself. Yet such interventions are by no means rare. Rarely are they therapeutic. A more appropriate approach may be to explore the expressed feeling in order to understand more fully the way in which the client is using words to describe feelings.

These, then, are some 'don'ts.' They are approaches to counselling interventions that are best avoided in that they are either heavily prescriptive, judgemental or inappropriate. As we have noted, there will be times when each is appropriate with this client at this point in time – particularly, perhaps, as the counselling relationship develops and counsellor and client get to know each other better.

QUESTIONS TO CONSIDER PRIOR TO COUNSELLING

Prior to commencing counselling, there are some questions that may usefully be considered in order to establish whether or not I am the appropriate person to counsel this person at this time.

Am I the appropriate person to counsel?

Sometimes we are too close to the person who comes to us for counselling. The concept of *therapeutic distance* is useful here. If we are emotionally too involved with the other person, we are probably too close to them to be able to stand back and assess their situation with reasonable objectivity. On the other hand, it is possible to stand too far back and be so detached from the other person that we are unable to appreciate their problems with any sensitivity at all. There would appear to be an optimum position in which to stand in relation to the client so that we are both disinterested and involved. Examples of people with whom we may be too involved include members of our family and close friends. Examples of people from whom we may be too distanced include (paradoxically) those people who present us with problems that are very similar to our own or who are so different from us that we fail basically to even empathize with them.

Have I the time to counsel?

Counselling takes time. At the outset, we may easily be able to afford the time we offer the client. This seems to be no problem when the client is initially depressed and it does not seem unreasonable to offer time. Once the client has begun to unravel some of his problems, the time factor becomes more pressing and it is remarkably easy to find that we are no longer sure that we have the time! It is important that we decide at the outset of the counselling relationship that we will be able to apportion adequate time for the other person. If we cannot, we should consider referring him to someone else.

On the other hand, there is much to be said for structuring the amount of time spent in counselling. It is useful to lay down clear time parameters as to the start and finish of the counselling session. It is often true that real client disclosure occurs towards the end of a counselling session – the important things are said last. If the client has no idea of when the session will end, he will clearly be unable to make these late and important disclosures. This issue of time will be discussed further in the next chapter.

Have I the client's permission to counsel?

Counselling is voluntary: no-one can be forced to disclose things that they are not ready or willing to disclose. On the other hand, it is easy to pressurize people into thinking that they should be counselled! When this happens, it is arguable that the counselling relationship is no longer a voluntary one: subtle coercion has taken place. It would seem better that it is always the client who seeks out the counsellor and never the counsellor who seeks out the client!

The term 'permission', as it is used here, is nearly always tacit permission: the fact that the client comes to the counsellor at all suggests that he gives permission for counselling to take place. Even when this initial, tacit contract has been established, however, it is important that the counsellor does not become intrusive and attempt to force disclosure where it is not freely offered. It is tempting, at times, for us to believe that disclosure will 'do the other person good'. This is an interesting value judgement but one that may say more about the counsellor's needs than those of the client!

Where will the counselling take place?

In an ideal world, counselling takes place on neutral territory: neither in the client's home nor in the office of the counsellor. Ideally, too, it is conducted in a room free from distractions, including other people who may knock on the door, telephones that may ring and surroundings that are so overstimulating that they distract the client's or counsellor's attention away from the task in hand. In practice, however, the environment is usually far removed from meeting these ideal criteria. Very often, counselling takes place wherever it occurs. Few people who work in the health professions can engineer the situation to such a degree that they can set up a particularly appropriate environment.

Having said that, there are environmental factors that may be borne in mind in almost all counselling settings. First, the chairs that both people sit in should be of the same height. This helps to create a certain equality in the relationship. If the counsellor sits at a higher or lower level than the client, it will be difficult for the relationship to develop. When the counsellor is sitting on a higher chair than the client, it puts her in a dominant position. When she is sitting on a lower chair, the relationship is such that the client is placed in a dominant position and may find this counterproductive to the telling of his story and to disclosing himself to the counsellor.

A further consideration is a seemingly odd one. It refers to where the counsellor and client sit in relation to the nearest window! It is difficult if either person sits with the window behind them (unless the lights are on!). If the counsellor sits with her back to the window, she will appear as a rather shadowy form because the client will be unable to see her properly. If the client sits in that position, the counsellor will not be able to see him properly and may miss vital aspects of non-verbal communication that can do much to convey particular thoughts and feelings. More suitable positions are well away from windows or ones in which both counsellor and client sit with the window to one side of them.

These are some important practical considerations that the health professional needs to consider before the specific skills of counselling are considered. Before such skills are discussed in detail, it may be useful to consider some basic principles of counselling that arise out of the literature and out of the discussion raised so far. These may be enumerated as follows.

1 The client knows what is best for him.
2 Interpretation by the counsellor is likely to be inaccurate and is best avoided.
3 Advice is rarely helpful.
4 The client occupies a different personal world from that of the counsellor and vice versa.
5 Listening is the basis of the counselling relationship.
6 Counselling techniques should not be overused; however,
7 counselling can be learned.

BASIC PRINCIPLES OF COUNSELLING

The client knows what is best for him or her

We all perceive the world differently as we all have different personal histories that colour our views. Throughout our lives we develop a variety of coping strategies that we use when beset by personal problems. Central to client-centred counselling, particularly, is the notion that, given the space and time, we are the best arbiters of what is and what is not right for us. We can listen to other people but in the end we, as individuals, have to decide upon our own courses of action.

Belief in the essential ability of all persons to make worthwhile decisions for themselves arises from the philosophical tradition known as existentialism (Macquarrie, 1973; Pakta, 1972). Existentialists argue, amongst other things, that we are born free and that we 'create' ourselves as we go through life. For the existentialist, nothing is predetermined: there is no blueprint for how any given person's life will turn out. Responsibility and choice lie squarely with the individual: we choose what we will become. Sartre (1973) sums up this position when he argues that:

> ***Man first of all exists, encounters himself and surges up in the world and defines himself afterwards. If man, as the existentialists see him, is not definable, it is because to begin with he is nothing. He will not be anything until later and then he will be what he makes of himself.***

No-one is free in all respects. We are born into a particular society, culture, family and body. On the other hand, our psychological make-up is much more fluid and arguably not predetermined. We are free to think and feel. One of the aims of the counselling relationship is to enable the client to realize this freedom to think and feel and, therefore, to act.

Once a person has to some extent recognized this freedom, he begins to realize that he can change his life. This is a central issue in the humanistic approach to counselling: that people can change (Shaffer, 1978). They do not have to be weighed down by the past or by their conditioning: they are more or less free to choose their own future. And no-one can choose that future for them. Hence the over-riding principle that the client knows what is best for them.

Interpretation by the counsellor is likely to be inaccurate and is best avoided

To interpret, in this sense, is to offer the client an explanation of his thinking, feeling or action. Interpretations are useful in that they can help us to clarify and offer a framework on which the client may make future decisions. However, they are best left to the client to make.

As we have seen, we all live in different perceptual worlds. Because of this, another person's interpretation of my thinking, feeling or action will be based on that person's experience, not mine. That interpretation is, therefore, more pertinent to the person offering it than it is to me, coloured as it is bound to be by the perceptions of the other person. Such colouring is usually more of a hindrance than a help. Often, too, interpretations are laced with moral injunctions – oughts and shoulds. Thus, an interpretation can quickly degenerate into moralistic advice that may lead to the client feeling guilty or rejecting the advice because it does not fit in with his own belief or value system.

Advice is rarely helpful

Attempts to help 'put people's lives right' are fraught with pitfalls. Advice is rarely directly asked for and rarely appropriate. If it is taken, the client tends to assume that 'That's the course of action I would have taken anyway' or he becomes dependent on the counsellor. The counsellor who offers a lot of advice is asking for the client to become dependent. Eventually, of course, some of the advice turns out to be wrong and the spell is broken: the counsellor is seen to be 'only human' and no longer the necessary lifeline perceived by the client in the past. Disenchantment quickly follows and the client–counsellor relationship tends to degenerate rapidly. It is better, then, not to become an advice giver in the first place.

There are exceptions to this principle where giving advice is appropriate – advice about caring for wounds, taking medication and health education, for example. In the sphere of personal problems, however, giving advice is rarely appropriate. Sartre (1973) notes, with some irony, that we tend to seek out people who we think will give us a certain sort of advice, the sort that we would tend to give ourselves! A further indication, perhaps, that it is better to enable the client to formulate their own advice rather than our supplying it.

The client and counsellor live in different 'personal worlds'

The fact that we have had varied experiences, have different physiologies and differing belief and value systems means that we perceive the world through different frames of reference. We tend to act according to our particular belief about how the world is. What happens next, however, is dependent upon how the world really is. If there is a considerable gap between our personal theory of the world and how the world actually is, we may be disappointed or shocked by the outcome of our actions. We may experience *dissonance* between what we believe to be the cause and what actually is.

It is important that the counsellor realizes that her own belief system may not be shared by the client and that the client may not see the world as she does. This is a basic starting point for the development of empathy in the relationship. To try to enter the frame of reference of the client accurately is one of the most important aspects of the relationship. It may also be one of the hardest, for we are always being invaded by our own thoughts, feelings, beliefs and values as we counsel.

A useful starting point is for the counsellor to explore her own belief and value systems before she starts. Simon *et al.* (1978) offer a series of useful exercises in values clarification. It is often surprising how contradictory and inconsistent our belief and value systems are! Once we are able to face some of these contradictions, we may be better able to face the contradictions in the client.

The counsellor's task is to attempt to enter and share the personal world of the client. That view usually changes as counselling progresses (Rogers and Dymond, 1978), after which the client may no longer feel the need for the counsellor. When this happens, the counsellor must develop her own strategies for coping with the separation that usually follows. Counselling is a two-way process. While the client's personal world usually changes, so may the counsellor's. The counselling relationship can, then, be an opportunity for growth and change for the counsellor as well as for the client.

Listening is the basis of the counselling relationship

To really listen to another person is the most caring act of all and takes skill and practice. Often when we claim to be listening, we are busy rehearsing our next verbal response, losing attention and failing to hear the other person. Listening involves giving ourselves up completely to the other person in order to fully understand them.

We cannot listen properly if we are constantly judging or categorizing what we hear. We must learn to set aside our own beliefs and values and to suspend judgement. We must also learn to develop *free-floating attention* – the ability to listen to the changing ebb and flow of the client's verbalizations and not to rush to pull them back to a particular topic. In this sense, what the client is talking about now is what is important. It is a process of offering free attention, of accepting totally the other person's story, accepting that their version of how the world is may be different from but just as valid as our own.

We need to listen to the metaphors, the descriptions, the value judgements and the words that the client uses: they are all indicators of their personal world. So, too, are facial expressions, body movements, eye contact (or lack of it) and other aspects of non-verbal communication.

Counselling techniques should not be overused

If we arm ourselves with a whole battery of counselling techniques, perhaps learned through workshops and courses, we may run into problems. The counsellor who uses too many techniques may be perceived by the client as artificial, cold and even uncaring. Perhaps we have all encountered the neophyte counsellor whose determined eye contact and stilted questions make us feel distinctly uncomfortable! It is possible to pay so much attention to techniques that they impede listening and communication.

Some techniques, such as the use of questions, reflections, summary, probing and so forth, are very valuable. They must, however, be used discretely and the human side of the counsellor must show through the techniques at all times. In the end, the quality of the relationship is more important than any techniques that may be used.

Counselling can be learned

Counselling, arguably, is something that comes naturally to some and not to others. We can all develop listening skills and the ability to communicate clearly with other people, which is the basis of effective counselling. The skills can be learned through personal experience and lots of practice, which may be gained in experiential learning workshops for the development of counselling skills and through the actual process of doing counselling.

The list of principles offered here is not exhaustive. It attempts to identify some of the important principles involved and to explain them. The next task will be to consider the process of the counselling relationship and to identify some of the stages that the relationship passes through as the client explores his world.

THE CULTURAL PERSPECTIVE IN COUNSELLING

There is an important cultural aspect to counselling which needs to be considered. Counselling can be thought of, in many ways, as an *individualistic* activity in which one person helps the other person to focus on their problems. Thus, the client's problems are viewed, mostly, as being tied up with their own responsibility for those problems and with their own ability to do something about them. Such an idea works in some cultures but not in others.

It is sometimes useful to make a distinction between *individualist cultures* and *collectivist cultures*. In individualist cultures, the person is seen as a discrete entity, with their own life, aspirations, hopes, wants and needs. The aim of the individual is often to strive to do better and to achieve more. In collectivist cultures, it is more usual to view the person as part of a group. In such cultures, it is usual not simply to focus on one person when problems occur but to involve the family or even the larger community. Indeed, in some cultures, particularly those in which certain religious beliefs predominate, it is seen as inappropriate to talk to another person, outside the family group, about 'personal' issues. In such cultures, too, there is not necessarily any sense of a need to strive towards personal goals nor to 'self-actualize' in any sense. Problems, when they occur, are resolved (or not resolved) within the family or local group. In a sense, counselling, and in particular client-centred counselling, is very much part of what used to be called a Western culture*. It focuses squarely on the individual and their difficulties. This would not necessarily work well within, for example, a Muslim culture or amongst the Maori population of New Zealand, which might be described as collectivist cultures. In Muslim cultures, it is far more likely that a person would go to a religious advisor to seek help about their problems and that the advice they are given would arise out of religious writings.

The role of the family and of elders varies very much from culture to culture and, in many, the older the person, the more respect they accrue. 'Courtesy' and even 'filial piety' are viewed as very positive qualities in many cultures. Most importantly, as indicated above, the individual is not everything in every culture.

In considering cultural issues, too, it is helpful to become aware of differences in non-verbal behaviours across different cultures. In many Buddhist and Muslim cultures, for example, there are a range of behaviours which are not usually seen as appropriate. Crossing of legs, pointing at another person with a finger, the use of direct eye contact, the touching of another person's head, whether or not people shake hands and, if they do, the strength and length of the handshake are just a few of the variants of non-verbal behaviours which are or are not acceptable in different cultural settings. The health care professional from Northern Europe or North America, when working in culturally diverse settings, would do well to learn more about these cultural differences. Otherwise, there is a danger of a sort of 'counselling imperialism' being generated in which health care professionals, training in counselling skills, come to think that their view of the world, of personal beliefs and of behaviours is somehow the 'right' one. In an important book about cultural differences in communication, McLaren (1998) offers, amongst others, the following suggestions.

1 Realize that cultural differences exist and matter. The assumption that underneath we are all the same can lead to all sorts of trouble. Misunderstandings occur not because communicators have different cultural orientations, but because they assume they share the same orientations and so misinterpret messages from each other.
2 Read about, observe and interact with people of other cultures so that you can recognize cultural differences and their meanings. Even in the very first meeting these may be crucial. Expect first meetings to be very formal, often through an intermediary and primarily intended to establish trust.

* There are, of course, difficulties in talking about 'Western' and 'Eastern' cultures as both are dependent upon the geographical position in which the speaker or writer is situated. For example, Australia seems, on the surface, to have much in common with the UK and the USA. However, it would be difficult to talk of it as being a 'Western' country, in the traditional sense of that term. This has become more of an issue as Australia seeks greater independence from the UK. Similarly, the terms 'occidental' and 'oriental' now seem patronizing and inappropriate to many people. It raises the question of why we *need* to separate out the world into two different areas in this way. The answer, I suspect, lies in political and economic theory.

3 Watch for unfamiliar and subtle signs of respect and formality which may be very different from those you are used to. Asking how old you are, for instance, may be a way of showing deference.
4 When you are perplexed about the way someone from another culture has reacted to a situation, consider the matter not from the point of view of the individual concerned but from that of the group to which he or she belongs. And remember that groups are flexible in an individualist culture but relatively fixed in a collective culture.

The matter of crosscultural counselling is a difficult and important one, particularly as health professionals work in increasingly diverse settings and as they take their skills to other countries. Anyone working in a very different culture from their own will need time to be absorbed into that culture and to understand or appreciate its mores. One of the most important issues in such integration is, of course, learning the language, for many cultural issues are mediated through verbal communication. However, as briefly indicated here, many are also mediated through sometimes complex non-verbal behaviours. Anyone who spends even a little time in a culture very different from their own soon becomes aware of the potential differences and difficulties of communication. Nor does the cultural setting necessarily *appear* to be so different: it is possible for an Australian to experience culture shock in the UK and for a British person to experience it in the USA. The fact that a given culture 'looks' the same as one's own is no real indicator of whether or not it is.

BASIC PRINCIPLES AND CONSIDERATIONS IN COUNSELLING IN THE HEALTH CARE PROFESSIONS

The degree to which the issues identified previously will fit with a particular health profession will vary according to the nature of the role of those professionals. For the physiotherapist, for example, the need to give clear and exact information may often be more of a priority than talking through emotional problems. For the nurse working with elderly people, listening to relatives may play a large part in the overall caring role. Given the different sorts of professional relationships that abound in the professions, it is important to modify the principles discussed in this chapter accordingly. Having said that, the principles apply fairly broadly to almost all relationships in one way or another. They need to be linked, also, to the maps of the counselling relationship discussed in the next chapter and the counselling skills outlined in the following chapters.

5 MAPS OF THE COUNSELLING RELATIONSHIP

Two counselling relationships can never be the same. We all come to counselling, whether as counsellor or as client, from different backgrounds and life experiences. Having said that, it may be helpful to sketch out in broad detail the possible nature of a typical counselling relationship. To this end, we need a *map* that can help us to explore the changing course of what happens between counsellor and client. Like any map, it is never the same as the territory itself. If we consider, for instance, the map of the London Underground system, it bears no geographical relationship to the actual layout of the rail network. More importantly, though, it gets us around London! So it may be with a map of the counselling process. I may never match exactly what happens in counselling, but it can help me to move through the relationship with greater ease.

Three different sorts of maps are offered here. The first is an eight-stage model that considers the changing and developing nature of the relationship. The second offers a very practical method of structuring the counselling process. The third considers three dimensions of counselling as a means of evaluating the relationship as it develops. The three can be used in various ways. First, one can be chosen as a way of working in counselling – the map chosen by the counsellor as the preferred one to be used in everyday practice, rather in the way that a person may use an AA map in preference to an Ordnance Survey map. Alternatively, any combination of the three may be used to highlight different aspects of counselling. The first, for example, may give a general overview of the whole relationship. The second may offer a practical set of steps that can be worked through. The third may highlight various aspects of counselling work that must be considered at various points throughout the relationship. The maps are not mutually exclusive: they all relate to the same thing and can be used together.

AN EIGHT-STAGE MAP OF THE COUNSELLING RELATIONSHIP

The stages in the model are enumerated below. It is suggested that this model offers a broad overview of how the relationship, typically, will unfold. Not all relationships will necessarily pass through each of the stages: some will reach certain stages and not others. Other relationships will bypass certain of the stages. The aim of the map is to offer a broad overview of the sorts of potential stages that many relationships will move through.

Stage one:meeting the client
Stage two:discussion of surface issues

Stage three:revelation of deeper issues
Stage four:ownership of feelings and, possibly, emotional release
Stage five:generation of insight: the client's life is viewed by them in a different light
Stage six:problem solving, future planning
Stage seven:action by the client
Stage eight:disengagement from the counselling relationship by the client

Stage one: meeting the client

In this first stage, the client meets the counsellor for the first time. Each is sounding out the other and setting tacit ground rules for the relationship. In a sense, both client and counsellor are 'on their best behaviour'. This is an important part of the larger counselling relationship in that it sets the tone for the whole dialogue. The skilled counsellor will set the client at ease in this stage and encourage him to gently spell out his reasons for talking to the counsellor. It is likely that both parties will experience some anxiety in this phase of the relationship: the client will want to be seen in a good light by the counsellor and the counsellor will be keen to ensure that the client feels comfortable in her company.

Stage two: discussion of surface issues

As the relationship slowly unfolds, the client will begin to tell his story or identify his problems in living. These will usually start with 'safe' disclosures: the deeper issues will reveal themselves later. Murray Cox (1978) offers a useful device for identifying the level of disclosure in the counselling relationship. He distinguishes between three levels of self-disclosure by the client: first, second and third levels. First-level disclosures are safe and relatively unimportant disclosures. First-level disclosures will vary according to the context but examples may be:

It took me a long time to get here today.
It took me a long time to find your office.
I haven't been to this part of the town before.

These are usually fairly polite statements that act as 'feelers' in relationship. They serve to test out the relationship in terms of trust and confidence. As the relationship deepens, so the level of self-disclosure increases. Levels two and three of Cox's model are in the following stage.

Stage three: revelation of deeper issues

Level two of Cox's (1978) model refers to the disclosure of feelings. Again, such disclosures will depend on the individual and the context but examples of such second-level disclosures may be:

I feel really angry about that.
I find it very difficult to feel positive about anything.
I'm not happy when I'm at home.

Second-level disclosures will not occur until the relationship between counsellor and client is sufficiently developed to the point where the client feels confident and trusting with the counsellor. It is a significant indicator that the relationship has deepened when the client begins to offer disclosure of how he is feeling.

Third-level disclosures are those that indicate the really deep, existential concerns of the client – the sorts of things that they may not have disclosed to any other person. If you stop reading for a moment and think of two things that very few people know about you, those would be third-level disclosures if you revealed them to another person. A clear principle emerges here: the client's potential third-level issues are not necessarily the same as the counsellor's third-level issues and vice versa. There is considerable danger in being misunderstood and in misunderstanding if we forget this. There is a temptation to believe that what troubles us is what troubles most people.

On the other hand, certain paradox arises here, for as Rogers (1967) notes: 'What is most personal is most general'. Some of the most difficult things to talk about turn out to be difficult for all of us. There is a certain commonality of human experience in that we all share certain fundamental difficulties. However, we should not assume that what I as a counsellor worry about, my clients worry about. Identification with the client is perhaps the most difficult issue here. We must be careful to draw the boundaries between ourselves and the client if we are to allow him to express his own third-level issues in his own time. It is arguable, too, that we will not allow the client to make third-level disclosures until we are accepting enough and comfortable with ourselves. We can easily and unconsciously put the client in the position of not being able to make these profound disclosures by our being defensive. To really listen to another person talking of their deeper human concerns is often a difficult business. This is yet another reason why we should, as counsellors, develop self-awareness; it may be only when we have faced some of our own third-level problems that we will allow the client to discuss his.

Third-level disclosures are often heralded by certain changes in the client. He may become more quiet, his facial expression may change and eye contact may be less sustained. If the person is saying something that has taken him considerable courage to disclose, that disclosure is bound to be accompanied by considerable anxiety. Often, if the counsellor sits quietly and attentively, the client will make the disclosure. If the counsellor is too talkative or questioning, the disclosure may be avoided all together. The timing of third-level disclosures by the client is fairly critical and if the circumstances of the relationship are not optimal and the disclosure has been made, often all that is necessary is for the counsellor to sit and listen to the client as he struggles to make sense of what has happened. Little intervention is needed at this point and the counsellor should avoid the temptation to 'overtalk' the client because of her own anxiety at being offered the disclosure (Heron, 1986).

Examples of typical third-level disclosures are difficult to describe.

More than any other sort, they tend to be idiosyncratic and defined by the context of the relationship. Many are metaphorical in nature. For example, the client may say: 'I never really had a childhood' or 'I realize that I have never felt anything really'. Others are more direct:

I've never loved my wife.
I hated my parents more than anything else.
I'm homosexual.

Third-level disclosures do not occur all together: they tend to be made at various points throughout the counselling relationship. Figure 5.1 demonstrates what may be termed the *rhythm of counselling* – the cycle of disclosures that starts with level one, deepens to level two and deepens still further to level three. It then, typically, lightens again and the client gradually returns to less difficult topics. Then the cycle starts again and the relationship deepens again. It may be important that this changing of level from deeper to lighter occurs. Too much disclosure, too quickly, can lead to the client feeling embarrassed and very deep disclosure made much too quickly can lead to the client returning only to first-level disclosures, never to revisit the more profound issues. Indeed, such sudden deep disclosure may lead to the client's subsequent withdrawal from the relationship altogether. Having made this very sudden disclosure, the client leaves feeling embarrassed and finds it difficult to return to face the counsellor again.

If such sudden, deep disclosure seems imminent at the beginning of a counselling relationship, it is sometimes sensible to lighten the

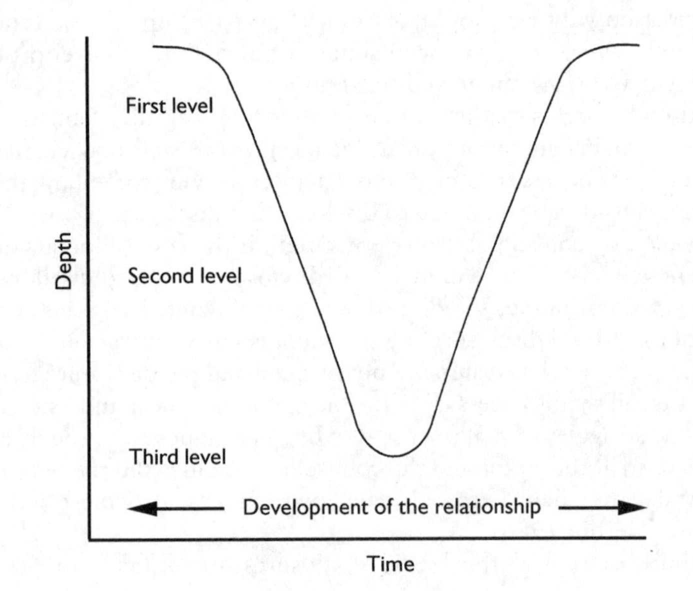

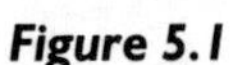
Figure 5.1

The rhythm of counselling (based on Cox, 1978).

conversation and allow the disclosure rate to slow down. In this way, the client discloses more gently and will feel more comfortable in the following sessions.

Third-level disclosures would seem to be an important part of the counselling process. The very fact that a client can articulate some of his deeper fears, anxieties and problems means that the possibility of resolving them is more likely. Also, the process of self-disclosure can often serve to change the client's perceptions of his problems. A considerable amount of energy is taken up with holding onto these more profound problems and the disclosure of them is often accompanied by a great sense of relief.

Clearly, third-level disclosures need to be received and heard by the counsellor with great tact. It is important that the client does not feel patronized or judged after such a disclosure. The very process of disclosure itself has been difficult enough, without the counsellor making the person feel more uncomfortable. As we have seen, the counsellor is often required to do nothing but listen. Also, too, the disclosure may be followed by a period of silence on the part of the client as he pieces together his thoughts on what he has said.

Stage four: ownership of feelings and possible emotional release

When the client has begun to talk about the very profound problems of his life, the tone of the dialogue will often change in a very significant way. The client stops talking about the feelings that he has in a general or detached sort of way and begins to experience the feelings themselves. In other words, the feelings begin to accompany the conversation. This can be described as *ownership* of those feelings. An example of the change in emotional state is illustrated in the following passage:

> 'Sometimes . . . sometimes when I'm at home, I get quite angry with various members of the family . . .' and 'Something odd is happening . . . I'm feeling angry now . . . I'm really furious! I won't be treated like that! It's my son, David . . . I'm really mad with him . . .'

The change can be quite dramatic as the client begins to thaw out and experience the feelings that he may have been bottling up for a considerable period. Sometimes the switch to experiencing the feelings as they are talked about is only transitory and the client quickly switches back to the safety of talking in the abstract. Sometimes, however, the sense of experiencing the feeling leads to more profound release of emotion, through tears, anger or fear – cathartic release. Sometimes, too, the embarrassment of the sudden realization of feeling leads to expression of that feeling in the form of laughter (Heron, 1989). This embarrassed laughter may quickly tip over into tears, anger or fear. Again, the counsellor's role is to allow the expression of feelings, the cathartic release. The tears, anger or fear may last for a few moments or may be sustained. The longer the counsellor can refrain from jumping to rescue the client from their feelings, the more likely it is that the client will benefit from the release.

Stage five: generation of insight: the client's life is viewed by them in a different light

It would seem that cathartic release generates insight (Heron, 1977b). If we can allow the expression of pent-up feeling and not interrupt the expression or attempt to interpret it, the client will come to view their life situation differently. It is as though the expression of pent-up feeling releases in the client a natural ability to think more rationally and see things more clearly. Often, all that is required in this stage is to sit quietly as the client experiences that insight. The client will not necessarily verbalize the insights gained through cathartic release but their non-verbal behaviour will usually indicate that the client is piecing the insights together. Often they will sit looking away from the counsellor, clearly thinking deeply. The temptation is often to interrupt that process with a series of questions but as a general rule, the process is best left undisturbed. The gain in insight is usually greater if the client can be allowed the time and space to appreciate it.

Stage six: problem solving and future planning

The expression of pent-up emotions and the insight gained through its release are not enough in themselves. The client still has to consider ways in which he is going to use that insight to change certain aspects of his life. Thus, once the tears have been shed and the perceptual shift has occurred, the client is often helped by the use of a practical problem-solving cycle (Burnard, 1985). Figure 5.2 offers one such cycle. In phase one, the problem is clearly defined by talking through the client's situation carefully and

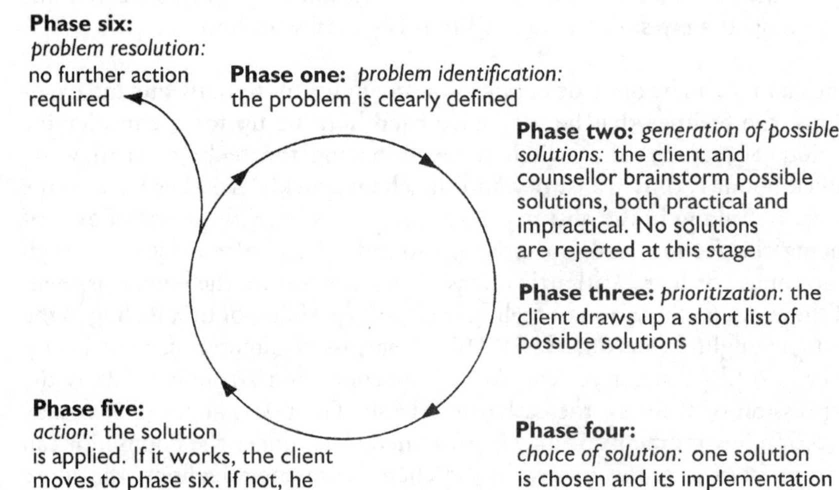

Figure 5.2

A problem-solving cycle.

helping them to express what they see as the problem as concisely as they can. In the second phase, the client and the counsellor generate as many possible solutions to that problem as they can. This process is sometimes known as brainstorming and involves considering every possibility, both rational and sensible and the more bizarre! Such a process can open up a fruitful and creative series of possible solutions that a plainly logical approach may not.

In phase three, a shortlist of possible solutions is drawn up and in stage four, the client makes a decision about which solution he will choose. Next, the solution is put into operation in the client's life and, if it works, the problem is resolved. If it does not, the problem-solving cycle can be worked through again, perhaps with a clearer definition of the problem.

Stage seven: action

As we noted at the outset, counselling must have a practical end. As the client comes to identify his problems of living, talk them through with the counsellor, express pent-up emotion and identify solutions, it is important that he introduces changes in his life. Indeed, if no such changes take place, the counselling is of very little use. This action stage of the relationship takes place away from the counsellor–client meetings and consists of the client trying new ways of living. During this stage, the client will obviously need a considerable amount of support from the counsellor but essentially, this will be the client's independent aspect of the relationship. It will also involve a growing independence on the part of the client who comes to realize that they can live without the counsellor and can make life choices without the counsellor's help. This stage shades into the next.

Stage eight: disengagement from the counselling process

This is what it says. Gradually, or sometimes abruptly, the client feels more and more able to cope on his own. Thus, the counselling relationship comes to an end. This may create considerable anxieties in both parties. The relationship has developed into a close one and to some degree, both people have become dependent on each other. The skilled counsellor is one who can effectively help in the disengagement process and not require the client to remain attached to her. This is the ultimate act of altruism, perhaps. It is the process of saying goodbye, with no strings attached. The goodbye must be unequivocal and without regret or remorse. The counsellor has completed her task and the client has learned to live for himself and with himself. Often, old issues of separation come to the fore, here. Bowlby (1975) wrote of 'separation anxiety' – the anxiety some people feel when they find a relationship coming to an end. Bowlby hypothesized that such people had experienced difficulties in early separations, in childhood or even in early infancy. Here, again, we find the need for the counsellor's developing self-awareness and the need for her to explore any identified difficulties with separations and with the ends of counselling relationships. It is important that such partings are smooth and that both parties are comfortable with the ending.

Reflecting on counselling

Can you be a counsellor and a personal friend to the client? Should you know the client 'outside' the professional relationship? This issue involves a considerable number of ethical issues which anybody setting out in counselling should consider.

A THREE-STAGE MODEL OF THE COUNSELLING RELATIONSHIP

The second map for guidance in the process of counselling is Egan's (1990) three-stage model of the helping relationship. His three stages are:

1. identifying and clarifying problem situations;
2. goal-setting: developing and choosing preferred scenarios;
3. action: moving towards the preferred scenario.

In stage one, the counsellor helps the client to tell his story, to explore his present life situation as he sees it now. Out of that story emerges the specific problems of living that could not have been identified prior to this exploratory process. It is as if the very telling of the story brings out the problems and puts a name to them. Egan notes also that this stage is useful for exploring 'blind spots' – aspects of the client's life that he had not considered.

In stage two, the client is helped to imagine a possible future situation that would be preferable to the present one. Initially, this often means imagining a variety of possible future scenarios, out of which the client slowly homes in on one. Once this realistic scenario has been discussed, the client and counsellor can identify goals that can help in the achievement of the proposed future state.

In stage three, the client and counsellor devise ways in which the proposed future scenario is achieved. In the first instance, this can be aided by the process of brainstorming, as described above. All possible methods of achieving the desired outcome are identified and then, gradually, a particular approach is chosen out of all the possibilities. Then, an action plan is drawn up in order to aid the achievement of the desired scenario further. The final substage of stage three is action on the part of the client – the time when the client makes the discussion concrete and puts the plan into action, supported by the counsellor.

Egan's (1986) three-stage model can serve as a useful and practical map in counselling and a means of bringing structure to the process of counselling. The three stages, although inter-related, can be dealt with as separate aspects of counselling and thus the relationship takes shape and has specific goals. Keeping the three stages in mind can help the counsellor to assess where the relationship is going and how it is developing. Obviously, no time limit can be put on how long each of the stages may take to work through with any given person but using them can ensure that the relationship remains dynamic and forward moving.

Egan's model in practice

June is an occupational therapist working with a group of young patients in a small psychiatric day hospital. She is approached by one patient, Alice, a girl recently discharged from hospital where she was treated for anorexia nervosa. Alice says that she wants to talk but is unclear about what her problems are. June uses Egan's three-stage model and allows Alice to describe everything that is happening to her at the present time. Thus, a picture of Alice's life emerges. Out of this picture, Alice identifies two problem areas: her overdependent relationship with her mother and her lack of self-confidence. June asks her to clarify how she would like the future to be. Alice talks of greater independence from her mother and an enhanced ability to socialize and mix more easily.

Out of their discussion, June and Alice draw up a list of practical, manageable tasks for the immediate future, including:

1. *Alice to set aside time to talk to her mother;*
2. *Alice to consider the practicality of finding a flat or bedsitter near parents' home;*
3. *Alice and June to work out a social skills training programme for Alice to follow with a group of other day hospital clients;*
4. *Alice to attend a weekend workshop on assertiveness training at a local college.*

THREE DIMENSIONS OF THE COUNSELLING RELATIONSHIP

Yet another way of mapping the relationship is in terms of three dimensions: time, depth and mutuality (Cox, 1978). Again, although each dimension overlaps with and is dependent on the others, each may be considered separately.

Time

The concept of time in the counselling relationship can be understood in at least two ways. First, there is the logical structuring of the counselling relationship itself. It makes sense for the counsellor to suggest a well-defined period of time for the counsellor–client meeting. Setting a boundary in this way has many advantages: once set, it can be forgotten about by both counsellor and client. Both know how long they will be together and when the session will finish. In an open-ended session, both may be confused about how long the session will last. A stated contract of, say, an hour overcomes this problem. The contract also means that the client will tend to use the time available constructively. As we have already noted, the client will often disclose important information towards the end of the meeting. If he does not know when that end will come, he may never make the disclosure. Also, an unstructured session may be fine when the counsellor is not busy but when constraints of work mean that the counselling session has to be truncated, the client may feel rejected. On balance, then, it seems better to structure the time more formally at the outset.

A second, more subtle aspect of time structuring relates to the focus of the counselling in terms of past, present and future. These three aspects may be considered as follows.

- Past – the client's past, personal history.
- Present – the client's present situation and the present situation for the client and counsellor together.
- Future – the client's aspirations, plans and hopes for what is to come.

In counselling those with emotional or psychological problems, it may be useful to consider spending roughly equal time in discussing all three time zones.

Our past experience has much to do with how we view the present. Indeed, what we are in the present may be seen as having grown out of past experience. Both past and present experience will determine, to a greater or lesser extent, how we make use of the future. Some people seem to want to live in the past; perhaps it was more comfortable or acceptable. Others look forward to what may happen in the future and dismiss the past as irrelevant – so much 'water under the bridge'. Tomorrow will always be better than today. Both living in the past and living for the future are, perhaps, unrealistic. To live in the present, with a strong sense of both past and future, may be more useful and constructive.

A balanced counselling relationship may take into account all three of these aspects of time. The counsellor may want to ask how the present situation is affected by past events and how the client views the future, given the present climate. If past, present and future are addressed in roughly equal amounts, then the momentum of the relationship remains continuous. There is a sense of continuity running through the relationship.

Depth

The second dimension in this map is depth. This refers to the aspects of intimacy and personal disclosure in the relationship and it depends on the amount of time invested in it. Depth cannot be hurried. It evolves out of the feeling of trust engendered by the client–counsellor process, but it does seem to develop in a cyclical manner. At the beginning of the relationship (and at the beginning of each counselling hour), there is usually a discussion of superficial things (first-level disclosures). As the relationship and the hour develop, so the depth of the relationship increases (through second- and third-level disclosures). The client slowly reveals himself to the counsellor and discloses more and more. Towards the end of the relationship (and the hour), the atmosphere lightens and the counselling relationship moves once again to a more superficial note. Thus, Cox's (1978) three levels of disclosure may be used to assess the depth of the relationship, both on a session-to-session basis and from the point of a longer term relationship. The three levels that Cox describes are illustrated in Figure 5.3.

First-level disclosures	'Lightweight' and easy disclosures	Example 'It's warm today and I seem to be in a bit of a hurry about things.'
Second-level disclosures	Disclosures of feelings accompanied by the effect	Example 'I feel really angry. I mean, I feel angry now!'
Third-level disclosures	Deepest, existential disclosures, perhaps never made before	Example: 'I feel as though I have never really been loved or loved anyone in my life...'

Figure 5.3

Cox's three levels of disclosure.

Many factors determine the depth of the relationship. A short list would include the counsellor's ability to empathize with the client, the counsellor's range of skills, the personalities and temperaments of counsellor and client, the degree of 'match' between the two people and the prevailing moods of both people.

First-level disclosures are clearly the easiest to make: they may sometimes merely be conversation. At other times, they signal the move towards greater trust in the counsellor and greater depth in the relationship. Second-level disclosures usually indicate that the client is able to express themselves more fully at the level of feelings and, thus, also indicate a further level of trust in the counselling relationship. Third-level disclosures occur once a considerable amount of work has been done in the counselling relationship and once the client feels able to trust the counsellor with his or her deepest fears or feelings. Paradoxically, though, they may also occur, spontaneously, at any stage in the counselling relationship and may surprise both the client and the counsellor. It is also vital that the counsellor *hears* third-levels disclosures and does not miss them. Sometimes, they occur so quickly and so spontaneously that the counsellor is caught unawares and does not really take in the importance of what has been disclosed. Sometimes, though, such disclosures are heralded by the client clearly building up towards 'saying something important'. There may be non-verbal signs. The client's tone of voice may drop, eye contact may be lessened as the client builds up the courage to say what they may not yet have said to anyone else. We can take it as something of a compliment that another person trusts us sufficiently to share their thoughts and feelings with us at this level. Such disclosure does not, of course, happen in all counselling relationships nor with all people. There are those who find disclosure easier than others.

While the three-stage model of disclosure is not foolproof, it does offer some guidance as to the depth that is being experienced in the counselling relationship. A more detailed discussion of the Cox disclosure model is found above, within the debate about the eight-stage counselling model.

Mutuality

The third dimension of structure is mutuality. This refers to the client's and counsellor's shared relationship with each other. As we noted earlier (p. 77), Martin Buber referred to the 'I–thou' relationship, the natural unfolding of relationship between two people who know each other on a reasonably equal and intimate level. Carl Rogers (1967) described the process of emerging from what resembled a hypnotic trance at the end of the counselling session. This trancelike state reflects the close nature of the truly mutual client–counselor relationship. Everything outside the relationship is forgotten while the client and counsellor are together – a close bonding occurs.

How does such mutuality develop? Arguably, it arises out of shared experiences and self-disclosure (although limits to this are discussed above). The counselling relationship, far from being a one-way traffic of disclosure from the client to the counsellor, becomes a time when human experiences are pooled. This is not to say that the counsellor should burden the client with her own problems, but to acknowledge that 'disclosure begets disclosure' (Jourard, 1964). I feel more understood when the person to whom I am talking shares something of their own experience with me.

To encourage mutuality, the counsellor has to develop an open, non-defensive and transparent presentation of self. Rather than hiding behind a professional mask, they allow themselves to be seen as they are, warts and all! It is worth noting that professionals who allow themselves to make mistakes occasionally are generally sensed as far more approachable and human than are their highly skilled, perfect counterparts. It would seem that affability is a necessary prerequisite of good counselling.

If this mutuality is missing, then the counselling process will remain superficial. If the counsellor always presents a professional facade and never allows the client to know her, then mutuality cannot develop. Mutuality is a measure of both the depth of the relationship and the counsellor's commitment to the relationship. It develops out of the counsellor's life experience, ability to empathize, skill and genuine commitment to the task.

These, then, are three ways of mapping out the counselling relationship. They differ in approach and degree of detail and perhaps they will appeal to different sorts of counsellors. Whilst no map is essential to counselling, some structure can help the unfamiliar to look a little less frightening. It can also suggest the direction forward and, at best, counselling should always be a dynamic and evolving process, though at times – like life itself – it will become stuck! Often, it is these periods of being stuck that are some of the most important. If we can stay with the 'stuckness' and even abandon the map, the result for the client in the long term can be much more rewarding.

MAPS OF THE COUNSELLING RELATIONSHIP AND THE HEALTH PROFESSIONAL

What map a particular health professional chooses in order to bring structure to their counselling will depend to a degree on the time available and the nature of the relationship. Where time is limited and a reasonable amount of resolution of a problem must be achieved, Egan's (1990) three-stage model is excellent. It is practical, structured and allows both health professional and client to see where the relationship is going and how it is progressing. Those professionals concerned with longer term relationships may choose the first and third models described in this chapter, for they emphasize more the processes that occur in the development of the counselling relationship. None of the maps, however, is mutually exclusive. They may be used in conjunction with each other and combined with the use of effective counselling skills described in the following chapters.

6 COUNSELLING SKILLS I: ATTENDING AND LISTENING

Listening and attending are by far the most important aspects of the counselling process. Often, the best counselling is that which involves the counsellor only listening to the other person. Unfortunately, most of us feel that we are obliged to talk! If we can train ourselves to give our full attention to and really listen to the other person, we can do much to help them. First, we need to discriminate between the two processes: attending and listening.

ATTENDING

Attending is the act of truly focusing on the other person. It involves consciously making ourselves aware of what the other person is saying and of what they are trying to communicate to us. Figure 6.1 demonstrates three hypothetical zones of attention.

Zone one, in the diagram, represents having our attention fully focused 'outside' ourselves and on the environment around us or, in the context of counselling, on the client. When we have our attention fully focused 'out' in this way, we are fully aware of the other person and not distracted by our own thoughts and feelings.

There are some simple activities, borrowed from meditation practice, that can enhance our ability to offer this sort of attention. Here is a particularly straightforward one. Stop reading this book for a moment and allow your attention to focus on an object in the room: it may be a clock or a picture or a piece of furniture – anything. Focus your attention on the object and notice every aspect of it: its shape, its colour, its size and so forth.

<table>
<tr>
<td rowspan="2">ZONE ONE: attention out

When attention is focused in this zone, the counsellor is fully listening to the client and paying attention to all verbal and non-verbal cues.</td>
<td>ZONE TWO: attention in

When attention is focused in this zone, the counsellor is caught up with his/her own thoughts and feelings. Attention to the client is only partial.</td>
</tr>
<tr>
<td>ZONE THREE: attention focused on fantasy

When attention is focused in this zone, the counsellor is busy trying to work out theories about the client. Rather than giving full attention, he/she is interpreting what is going on.</td>
</tr>
</table>

Figure 6.1

Three possible zones of attention.

Continue to do this for at least one minute. Notice, as you do this, how your attention becomes fully absorbed by the object. You have focused your attention 'out'. Then discontinue your close observation. Notice what is going on in your mind. What are your thoughts and feelings at the moment? When you do this, you shift your attention to zone two, the 'internal' domain of thoughts and feelings. Now shift the focus of your attention out again and onto another object. Study every aspect of it for about a minute. Notice, as you do this, how it is possible to consciously shift the focus of your attention in this way. You can will yourself to focus your attention outside yourself. Practice at this conscious process will improve your ability to fully focus attention outside yourself and onto the client.

Clearly, if we are to pay close attention to every aspect of the client, it is important to be able to move freely between zones one and two. In practice, what probably happens in a counselling session is that we spend some time in zone one, paying full attention to the client and then we shuttle back into zone two and notice our reactions, feelings and beliefs about what they are saying, before we shift our attention back out. The important thing is that we learn to gain control over this process. It is no longer a haphazard, hit-and-miss affair but we can learn to focus attention with some precision. It is not until we train ourselves to consciously focus attention 'out' in this way that we can really notice what the other person is saying and doing.

Zone three in the diagram involves fantasy: ideas and beliefs that bear no direct relation to what is going on at the moment but to what we think or believe is going on. When we listen to another person, it is quite possible to think and believe all sorts of things about them. We may, for example, think 'I know what he's really trying to tell me. He's trying to say that he doesn't want to go back to work, only he won't admit it – even to himself!'. When we engage in this sort of 'internal dialogue' we are working within the domain of fantasy. We cannot 'know' other things about people unless we ask them or, as Epting puts it: 'If you want to know what someone is about, ask them – they may just tell you!' (Epting, 1984). We often think that we do know what other people think or feel, without checking with that person first. If we do this, it is because we are focusing on the zone of fantasy: we are engaged in the processes of attribution or interpretation. The problem with these sorts of processes is that, if they are wrong, we may develop a very distorted picture of the other person! Our assumptions naturally lead us to other assumptions and if we begin to ask questions directly generated by those assumptions, our counselling will lack clarity and our client will end up very confused!

A useful rule, then, is that if we find ourselves within the domain of fantasy and we are 'inventing' things about the person in front of us, we stop and if necessary check those inventions with the client to test the validity of them. If the client confirms them, all well and good: we have intuitively picked up something about the client that he was, perhaps, not consciously or overtly telling us. If, on the other hand, we are wrong, it is probably best to abandon the fantasy all together. The fantasy, invention or assumption probably tells us more about our own mental make-up than it does about that of our client! In fact, these 'wrong' assumptions can help us gain more self-awareness. In noticing the wrong assumptions we make about others, we can reflect on what those assumptions tell us about ourselves.

Awareness of focus of attention and its shift between the three zones has implications for all aspects of counselling. The counsellor who is able to keep attention directed out for long periods is likely to be more observant and more accurate than the counsellor who is not. The counsellor who can discriminate between the zone of thinking and the zone of fantasy is less likely to jump to conclusions about their observations or to make value judgements based on interpretation rather than fact.

What is being suggested here is that we learn to focus directly on the other person (zone one) with occasional moves to the domain of our own thoughts and feelings (zone two) but that we learn to attempt to avoid the domain of fantasy (zone three). It is almost as though we learn to meet the client as a 'blank slate': we know little about them until they tell us who they are. To work in this way in counselling is, almost paradoxically, much more empathic. We learn not to assume things about the other person but to listen to them and to check out any hunches or intuitions we may have about them.

Being able to focus on zone one and have our attention focused out has other advantages. In focusing in this way, we can learn to maintain the 'therapeutic distance' referred to in a previous chapter. We can learn to distinguish clearly between what are the client's problems and what are our own. It is only when we become mixed up by having our attention partly focused on the client, partly on our own thoughts and feelings and partly on our fantasies and interpretations that we begin to get confused about what the client is telling us and what we are 'saying to ourselves'. We easily confuse our own problems with those of the client.

Second, we can use the concept of the three domains of attention to develop self-awareness. By noticing the times when we have great difficulty in focusing attention 'out', we can learn to notice points of stress and difficulty in our own lives. Typically, we will find it difficult to focus attention out when we are tired, under pressure or emotionally distressed. The lack of attention that we experience can serve as a signal that we need to stop and take stock of our own life situation. Further, by allowing ourselves consciously to focus 'in' on zones two and three – the process of introspection – we can examine our thoughts and feelings in order to further understand our own make-up. Indeed, this process of self-exploration seems to be essential if we are to be able to offer another person sustained attention. If we constantly 'bottle up' problems we will find ourselves distracted by what the client has to say. Typically, when they begin to talk of a problem of theirs that is also a problem for us, we will suddenly find our attention distracted to zone two: suddenly we will find ourselves pondering on our own problems and not those of the client! Regular self-examination can help us to clear away, at least temporarily, some of the more pressing personal problems that we experience. A case, perhaps, of 'counsellor, counsel thyself!'

Such exploration can be carried out in isolation, in pairs or in groups. The skills exercises part of this book offers practical suggestions as to how such exploration can be developed. If done in isolation, meditative techniques can be of value. Often, however, the preference will be to conduct such exploration in pairs or groups. In this way, we gain further insight through hearing other people's thoughts, feelings and observations and we can make useful comparisons between other people's experience and our own. There are a variety of formats for running self-awareness groups, including sensitivity groups, encounter groups, groups therapy and training groups. Such groups are often organized by colleges and extramural departments of universities but they can also be set up on a 'do-it-yourself' basis. Ernst and Goodison (1981) offer some particularly useful guidelines for setting up, running and maintaining a self-help group for self-exploration. Such a group is useful as a means of developing self-awareness, as a peer support group for talking through counselling problems and also as a means of developing further counselling skills. Trying out new skills in a safe and trusting environment is often a better proposition than trying them out with real clients!

Attending in practice

Elizabeth, a health visitor, finds that during a busy day, it is difficult to 'cut off' from one client before visiting another. She finds herself preoccupied with the problems of a previous visit during a visit to another person. Through practising the process of focusing 'attention out' between visits and by taking a few minutes, in her car, to 'dissociate' from the client she has just visited, she develops the skill of giving full attention to the next person she sees.

LISTENING

Listening is the process of 'hearing' the other person. This involves, not only noting the things that they say but also a whole range of other aspects of communication. Figure 6.2 outlines some of the things that can be noted during listening.

Given the wide range of ways in which one person tries to communicate with another, this is further evidence of the need to develop the ability to offer close and sustained attention, as outlined above. Three aspects of listening are noted in the diagram. Linguistic aspects of speech refer to the actual words that the client uses, to the phrases they choose and to the metaphors they use to convey how they are feeling. Attention to such metaphors is often useful as metaphorical language can often convey more than conventional use of language (Cox, 1978). Paralinguistics refers to all those aspects of speech that are not words. Thus, timing, volume, pitch, and accent are all paralinguistic aspects of communication. Again, they can offer us indicators of how the other person is feeling beyond the words that

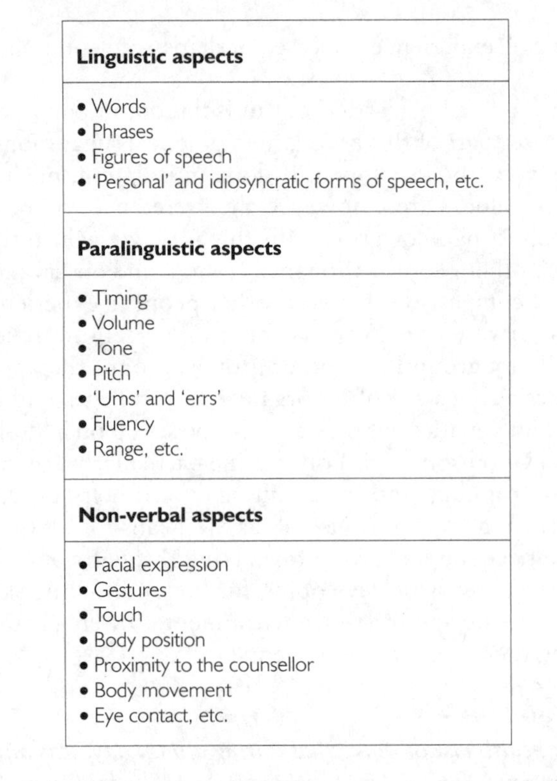

Figure 6.2

Aspects of listening.

they use. However, we must be careful of making assumptions and slipping into zone three, the zone of fantasy. Paralinguistics can only offer us a possible clue to how the other person is feeling. It is important that we check with the client the degree to which that clue matches with the client's own perception of the way they feel.

Non-verbal aspects of communication can be called 'body language': the way that the client expresses himself through the use of his body. Thus, facial expression, use of gestures, body position and movement, proximity to the counsellor, touch in relation to the counsellor, all offer further clues about the client's internal state and can be 'listened to' by the attentive counsellor. Again, any assumptions that we make about what such body language 'means' need to be clarified with the client. There is a temptation to believe that body language can be 'read', as if we all used it in the same sort of way. This is, perhaps, encouraged by works such as Desmond Morris's (1978) *Manwatching*. Reflection on the subject, however, will reveal that body language is dependent on many variables: the context in which it occurs, the nature of the relationship, the individual's personal style and preference, the personality of the person 'using' the body language, and so on. It is safer, therefore, not to assume that we 'know' what another person is 'saying' with their body language but again to, treat it as a clue and to clarify with the client what he means by his use of it. Thus, it is preferable to merely bring to the client's attention the way they are sitting or their facial expression, rather than to offer an interpretation of it. Two examples may help here. In the first, the counsellor is offering an interpretation and an assumption.

> I notice from the way that you have your arms folded and from your frown that you are uncomfortable with discussing things at home.

In the second example, the counsellor merely feeds back to the client what she observes and allows the client to clarify his situation.

> I notice that you have your arms folded and that you're frowning. What are you feeling at the moment?

LEVELS OF LISTENING

The skilled counsellor learns to listen to all three aspects of communication and tries to resist the temptation to interpret what she hears. Three levels of listening may be identified, as shown in Figure 6.3

The first level of listening refers to the idea of the counsellor merely noting what is being said. In this mode, client and counsellor are not psychologically very 'close' and arguably the relationship will not develop very much. In the second level of listening, the counsellor learns to develop free-floating attention: she listens 'overall' to what is being said, as opposed to trying to catch every word. Free-floating attention also refers to

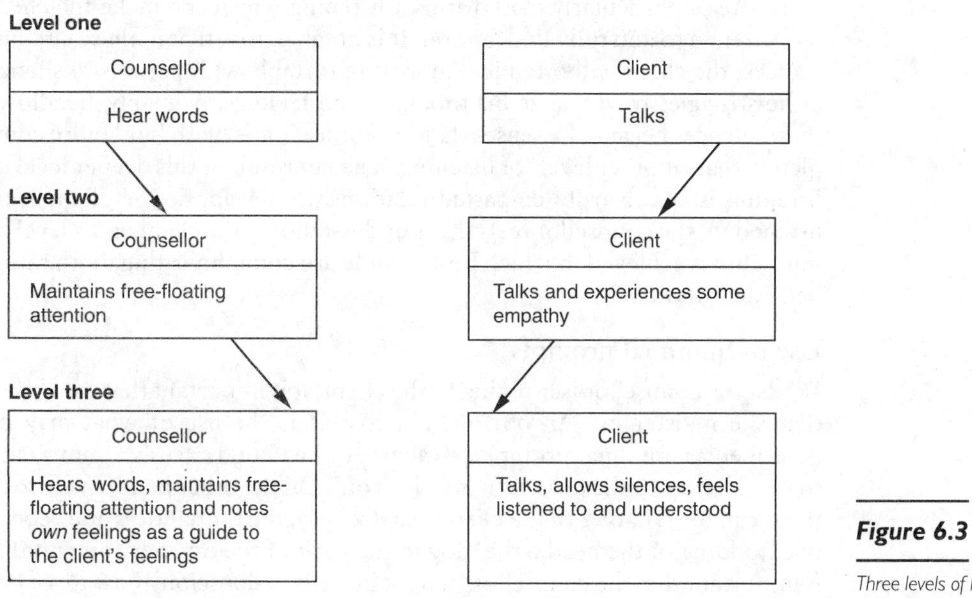

Figure 6.3

Three levels of listening.

'going with' the client, not trying to keep the client to a particular theme but following the client's conversation wherever it goes. She also 'listens' to the client's non-verbal and paralinguistic behaviour as indicators of what the client is thinking and feeling. Faced with this deeper level of listening, the client feels a greater amount of empathy being offered by the counsellor. The counsellor begins to enter the frame of reference of the client and to explore his perceptual world. She begins to see the world as the client experiences it.

In the third level of listening, the counsellor maintains free-floating attention, notices non-verbal and paralinguistic aspects of communication but also notices her own internal thoughts, feelings and body sensations. As Rollo May (1983) notes, once the counselling relationship has deepened, what the counsellor is feeling can be a direct mirror image of what the client is feeling. Thus, the counsellor sensitively notices changes in her self and gently checks these with the client. It is as though the counsellor is listening both to the client and to herself and carefully using herself as a sounding board for how the relationship is developing. Watkins (1978) has described this process as 'resonance' and points out that this process is different from that of empathizing.

> *Rogers says that empathy means understanding of the feelings of another. He holds that the therapist does not necessarily himself experience the feelings. If he did, according to Rogers, that would be identification, and this is not the same as empathy. Resonance is a type of identification which is temporary.*

The use of resonance needs to be judged carefully. Whilst it does not involve interpreting or offering a theory about what the client is feeling, it does offer a particularly close form of listening which can make the client feel listened to and fully understood. It is notable, too, that in these circumstances, the client will often feel more comfortable with periods of silence as he struggles to verbalize his thoughts and feelings. Arguably, he allows these silences because he senses that the counsellor is 'with him' more completely than at other levels of listening. The net result of this deeper level of listening is that a truly empathic relationship develops. The client feels listened to, the counsellor feels she is understanding the client and a level of mutuality is achieved in which both people are communicating, both rationally and intuitively.

Use of 'minimal prompts'

Whilst the counsellor is listening to the client, it is important that she shows that she is listening. An obvious aid to this is the use of what may be described as 'minimal prompts' – the use of head nods, 'yes's', 'mm's' and so on. All these indicate that 'I am with you'. On the other hand, overuse of them can be irritating to the client, particularly, the thoughtless and repetitive nodding of the head – the 'dog in the back of the car' phenomenon! It is important that the counsellor, at least initially, is consciously aware of her use of minimal prompts and tries to vary her repertoire. It is important to note, also, that very often such prompts are not necessary at all. Often, all the client needs is to be listened to and appreciates that the counsellor is listening, without the need for further reinforcement of the fact.

BEHAVIOURAL ASPECTS OF LISTENING

One other aspect of the process of listening needs consideration and that is the behaviours the counsellor adopts when listening to the client. Egan (1990) offers the mnemonic SOLER as a means of identifying and remembering the sorts of counsellor behaviour that encourage effective listening.

Sit Squarely in relation to the client,
maintain an Open position,
Lean slightly towards the client,
maintain reasonable Eye contact with the client,
Relax!

First, the counsellor is encouraged to sit squarely in relation to the client. This can be understood both literally and metaphorically. In North America and the UK it is generally acknowledged that one person listens to another more effectively if she sits opposite or nearly opposite the other person, rather than next to him. Sitting opposite allows the counsellor to see all aspects of communication, both paralinguistic and non-verbal, that might be missed if she sat next to the client. Second, the counsellor should consider adopting an open position in relation to the client. Again, this can be understood both literally and metaphorically. A 'closed' attitude is as much a block to effective counselling as is a closed body position. Crossed arms and legs, however, can convey a defensive feeling to the client and counselling is often more effective if the counsellor sits without crossing either. Having said that, many people feel more comfortable sitting with their legs crossed, so perhaps some licence should be used here! However, the counsellor should avoid sitting in a 'knotted' position with both arms and legs crossed.

It is helpful if the counsellor appreciates that they can lean towards the client. This can encourage the client and make them feel more understood. If this does not seem immediately clear, next time you talk to someone, try leaning away from the other person and note the result!

Eye contact with the client should be reasonably sustained and a good rule of thumb is that the amount of eye contact that the counsellor uses should roughly match the amount the client uses. It is important, however, that the counsellor's eyes should be 'available' for the client in that the counsellor is always prepared to maintain eye contact. On the other hand, it is important that the client does not feel stared at or intimidated by the counsellor's glare. Conscious use of eye contact can ensure that the client feels listened to and understood but not uncomfortable.

The amount of eye contact the counsellor can make will depend on a number of factors, including the topic under discussion, the degree of 'comfortableness' the counsellor feels with the client, the degree to which the counsellor feels attracted to the client, the amount of eye contact the client makes, the nature and quality of the client's eye contact and so forth. If the counsellor continually finds the maintenance of eye contact difficult it is, useful to consider talking the issue over with a trusted colleague or with a peer support group, for eye contact is a vital channel of communication in most interpersonal encounters (Heron, 1970).

Finally, it is important that the counsellor feels relaxed while listening. This usually means that she should refrain from 'rehearsing responses' in her head. It means that she gives herself up completely to the task of listening and trusts herself that she will make an appropriate response when she has to. This underlines the need to consider listening as the most important aspect of counselling. Everything else is secondary to it. Many people feel that they have to have a ready response when engaged in a conversation with another person. In counselling, however, the main focus of the conversation is the client. The counsellor's verbal responses, although important, must be secondary to what the client has to say. Thus all the counsellor has to do is to sit back and intently listen. Easily said but not so easily done! The temptation to 'overtalk' is often great but can lessen with more experience and with the making of a conscious decision not to make too many verbal interventions.

All these behavioural considerations can help the listening process. In order to be effective, however, they need to be used consciously. The counsellor needs to pay attention to using them and choose to use them. As we have noted, at first this conscious use of self will feel uncomfortable and unnatural. Practice makes it easier and with that practice comes the development of the counsellor's own style of working and behaving in the counselling relationship. No such style can develop if the counsellor does not first consciously consider the way she sits and the way she listens.

In summary, it is possible to identify some of those things which act as blocks to effective listening and some aids to effective listening. No doubt the reader can add to both of these lists and such additions will be useful in that they will be a reflection of your own strengths and limitations as a listener.

A note of caution

While the above paragraphs have stressed the need for the counsellor to be aware of their own non-verbal aspects of behaviour while listening, it can be overdone. It is important, perhaps, not to develop a 'counsellor's face' and exercise facial expressions and eye contact to such a degree that the client is very aware that the counsellor is using such behaviours. I recall that some years ago, after I had attended a number of counselling courses, I was with a friend who, as we sat and talked, suddenly said 'I'm being listened to!' and was clearly uncomfortable. Flannery O'Connor, in his short story *Good Country People*, describes this 'obvious' presentation of facial expression as follows.

> *Besides the neutral expression that she wore when she was alone, Mrs Freeman had two others, forward and reverse, that she used for all her human dealings. Her forward expression was steady and driving like the advance of a heavy truck. Her eyes never swerved to left or right but turned as the story turned as if they followed a yellow line down the centre of it. She seldom used the other expression because it was not often necessary for her to retract a statement, but when she did, her face came to a complete stop, there was an almost imperceptible movement of her black eyes, during which they seemed to be receding, and then the observer would see that Mrs Freeman, though she might stand there as real as several grain sacks thrown on top of each other, was no longer there in spirit. (O'Connor, 1998)*

We should be wary of becoming too obvious.

Blocks to effective listening

- The counsellor's own problems;
- counsellor stress and anxiety;
- awkward/uncomfortable seating;
- lack of attention to listening behaviour;
- value judgements and interpretations on the part of the counsellor;
- counsellor's attention focused 'in' rather than 'out';
- 'rehearsals' inside the counsellor's head.

While numerous conditions exist in which listening may be difficult, Egan (1990) offers a useful list of some possibilities that can make listening to another person a problem.

- *Attraction*. You find a client either quite attractive or quite unattractive. You pay more attention to what you are feeling about the client than to what the client is saying.
- *Physical condition*. You are tired or sick. Without realizing it, you tune out some of the things the client is saying.
- *Concerns*. You are preoccupied with your own concerns. For instance, you keep thinking about the argument you've just had with your spouse.
- *Overeagerness*. You are so eager to respond that you listen to only a part of what the client has to say. You become preoccupied with your responses rather than with the client's revelations.
- *Similarity of problems*. The problems the client is dealing with are quite similar to your own. As the client talks, your mind wanders to the ways in which what is being said applies to you and your situation.
- *Differences*. The client and their experience is very different from you and your experiences. This lack of communality is distracting.

Aids to effective listening

- Attention focused 'out';
- suspension of judgement by the counsellor;
- attention to the behavioural aspects of listening;
- comfortable seating;
- avoidance of interpretation;
- development of free-floating attention;
- judicious use of minimal prompts.

LISTENING: A SKILL OR A QUALITY?

In a recent study, I surveyed some health care students about their perceptions of the *qualities* of a good counsellor.

The term 'counsellor', in this case, was defined as 'the sort that a person might go to see to talk about personal or emotional problems'. This was to differentiate between a counsellor as helper and confidante and other sorts of counsellors such as coaches, information givers, trainers and supervisors.

Two hundred health care students, on a range of courses, were surveyed. Students could choose whether or not they completed the form. One hundred and sixty-two usable survey papers were returned – a response rate of 81%.

Respondents were asked to identify up to ten personal qualities that they might expect to find in a counsellor. They were given the following instructions.

> I am interested in your views about what you feel are the *personal qualities* that could reasonably be expected to be found in a counsellor. A 'counsellor' in this case is the sort that a person might go to see to talk about personal or emotional problems.
>
> I would be grateful if you would list, below, the personal qualities that *you* would expect to find in a counsellor. There are no right or wrong suggestions but please bear in mind that this study focuses on *qualities* and not on *skills* or *qualifications*. You can list as few qualities as you like but please list no more than ten.

Analysis of the data

Despite the request to list no more than ten qualities, a number of students identified more than ten. These other qualities were included in the analysis. The range of qualities identified by individual respondents was 3–15.

All the responses were listed in a word-processing file. These items were then placed in alphabetical order to facilitate frequency counting of the various items. From this list it was possible to manually count the number of occurrences, within the total sample, of various personal qualities identified by the students. Percentages were then calculated and the findings placed in rank order. Given the sampling method used, it was deemed inappropriate to use any form of inferential statistics on the data.

Findings

Among the most frequently identified qualities were those broadly in line with previous research and the literature: being non-judgemental, being empathic and understanding (Rogers, 1967; Egan, 1990; Burnard, 1995). However, other qualities such as being approachable, sympathetic and caring rated highly, too. Often, empathy is identified in the literature as an important personal quality where sympathy is not. However, these items represent abstractions and, as such, may be difficult to define clearly. Safety and ethical qualities also appeared to be important (such as being confidential, trustworthy and honest). It should be noted, too, that some respondents addressed the issue in terms of 'negatives' (e.g. counsellors should be non-threatening, non-patronizing or not forceful). The surprise 'quality', perhaps, was *good listener.* Seventy-three percent of the sample identified 'good listener' as a personal quality. As we shall see in the discussion below, this runs counter to much of the literature which defines listening as a skill rather than a quality. Figure 6.4 identifies the range of findings down to qualities identified by at least five respondents.

Discussion

The findings highlight an interesting ambiguity. Although the literature on counselling often identifies listening as a skill (see, for example, BAC 1989a, b; Davis and Fallowfield, 1991; Morrison and Burnard, 1997), many of the respondents in this study identified it as a personal quality. This is underlined by the facts that the researcher clearly indicated that he was interested only in personal qualities and not in skills, as discussed above, and that no other skills were identified in this way. If the respondents were generally mistaking or confusing qualities with skills, it would be likely that they would identify other skills in this way.

Thus, it would appear that, for these respondents at least, the issue of skills versus qualities merges when it comes to listening. This ambiguity is hinted at, but not made explicit, in a British Association for Counselling Code of Conduct which makes an apparent demarcation between 'listening skills' and 'counselling skills'.

> ***The term 'counselling skills' does not have a single definition which is universally accepted. For the purpose of this code, 'counselling skills' are distinguished from 'listening skills' and from 'counselling'. Although the distinction is not always a clear one, because the term 'counselling skills' contains elements of these two activities, it has its own place between them . . . (BAC, 1989a)***

Although the BAC is not particularly clear on the issue – partly, as it admits,

Quality	n	%
Good listener	119	73
Non-judgemental	93	57
Empathic	56	35
Understanding	56	35
Approachable	43	27
Sympathetic	32	20
Caring	31	19
Friendly	31	19
Patient	28	17
Confidential	27	17
Supportive	22	14
Knowledgeable	19	12
Honest	18	11
Trustworthy	16	10
Experienced	12	7
Kind	12	7
Warm	12	7
Calm	11	7
Helpful	9	6
Respectful	8	5
Sense of humour	8	5
Advice giving	7	4
Considerate	7	4
Genuine	7	4
Open	7	4
Open minded	7	4
Professional	7	4
Non-patronizing	6	4
Objective	6	4
Reassuring	6	4
Trusting	6	4
Broad minded	5	3
Comforting	5	3
Communicative	5	3
Relaxed	5	3

Figure 6.4

Qualities of counsellors as identified by students (n=162)

because the issue, in general is not clear – they hint at a distinction between listening skills and counselling skills as two, possibly discrete, categories. The present findings seem to argue against making such a clear distinction between 'listening', 'counselling skills' and 'personal qualities'. Listening, it would seem, may straddle a distinction between skills and personal qualities and leaves in the air the question: 'Is listening a skill or a quality?' For the moment, though, we should note that the BAC, in the quotation above, is still considering listening as a skill.

The question of whether or not listening is a skill or a personal quality is not easily answered and it may be noted that at least one writer offers a definition of listening that seems to indicate something more complex – and perhaps more personal – than mere skill.

> ***Listening is the complex, learned human process of sensing, interpreting, evaluating, storing and responding to oral messages. (Steil, 1991)***

It is notable, too, that in the study described here, an educator who also completed one of the survey forms commented as follows.

> ***Qualities are very difficult to differentiate from skills because the personal qualities of a counsellor are often conveyed through competence in skills such as listening, empathic responding, etc. etc.***

It would seem possible, then, that personal qualities may be mediated through the demonstration of certain skills. On the other hand, it seems quite possible to rote learn a range of skills and to *not* have the personal qualities behind those skills. The demonstration of skills does not offer conclusive evidence of particular qualities. The task of discerning underlying qualities or intentions from behaviour remains problematic.

The literature on counselling training often refers to the teaching of 'listening skills' (see, for example, Ellis and McClintock, 1994; Williams, 1997). The suggestion is that, given practice and appropriate educational experiences, students can enhance their listening through rehearsing the skill. However, if listening is considered a quality or, perhaps, a quality and a skill, such an approach might have to be modified. For, it might be argued, personal qualities are not the sorts of characteristics that can so readily be honed by training.

It would seem possible that listening is more than simply a collection of behaviours to be learned. It is likely, too, that listening, in a therapeutic sense, involves more than just hearing and acknowledging the words spoken by another person. Arguably, though, many of the methods used to teach 'listening skills' focus on behavioural elements of the process: on sitting in a certain way, on maintaining eye contact, on using minimal prompts, on paying attention to non-verbal cues and so on (Kagan *et al.*, 1986; Egan, 1990; Hobbs, 1992).

While these are likely to be valuable in helping people to focus during the listening process, they do not capture some of the more subtle aspects of listening. We might argue, in the light of listening being considered a personal quality, that listening also involves a more subjective, difficult to pin down aspect – perhaps akin to Martin Buber's notion of the meeting of two 'subjects' in the 'I–Thou' relationship (Buber, 1958).

One possible solution to the issue of what constitutes a counselling skill and what constitutes a personal quality is to use the term 'characteristic' in place of both. Thus we might talk of the 'characteristics of a counsellor' and that might include both skills and qualities. It is acknowledged, however, that this is perhaps a semantic 'fudge' and may only be a way of circumventing further debate on the importance, or otherwise, of the differences between human qualities and demonstrable skills. On the other hand, if we accept the point that 'personal qualities' may *not* play the major role in the counselling relationships and that skills are just as important, it may seem reasonable to merge the distinction between qualities and skills by the use of the term 'characteristic'.

This, in turn, may mean that some teachers of counselling skills to health care professionals may have to change their approach. Given the emphasis in the literature on 'counselling skills', the challenge may be to present the characteristics of an effective counsellor in ways that embrace both personal qualities and previously identified skills. Further, there might be discussion about whether or not it is possible to 'train' health care professionals in particular personal qualities. While listening remains a skill, it seems possible to engage in skills training. If listening is more than a skill and becomes a quality, then we may or may not be able to engage in 'qualities training'. Many people would claim that, by definition, personal qualities are more idiosyncratic and less visible than skills. Clearly, more work needs to be done to validate or reject the particular finding of this study.

ATTENDING, LISTENING AND THE HEALTH PROFESSIONAL

The attending and listening aspects of counselling are essential skills that can be used in every health professional's job. The skills are clearly not limited only to use within the counselling relationship but can be applied in other interpersonal exchanges. An advantage of paying attention to the development of these particular skills is that becoming an effective listener not only makes for better counselling practice but interpersonal effectiveness and self-awareness are also enhanced. In the following chapters, verbal interventions are explored that will complement the listening and attending described here. Again, such interventions can be used both inside and outside the counselling relationship and can do much to improve every health professional's performance as a carer.

Listening in practice

David is a GP in a busy city-centre practice. He gets repeated visits from a young woman, Sarah, whose husband has recently been killed in a road accident. She often makes allusion to the problems of adjusting to her bereavement but presents with fairly minor physical ailments. David gently suggests to her that it may be helpful if they talked about her loss in more detail and offers her a booked appointment. At first she is reluctant to accept this but later phones to make such an appointment. During the next few weeks, David meets Sarah on a regular basis and listens to her. During these appointments, he has to make very few verbal interventions: Sarah is able to describe and ventilate her feelings very easily, once she is offered the opportunity. She works through stages of anger, extreme sorrow and meaninglessness and finally to some acceptance. During these stages, David has had to 'do' very little. His supportive attention and ability to listen, without making too many suggestions or offering too much advice, has been therapeutic in itself. He realizes, however, that he has had to 'learn to listen'. Previously in his career, he tended to be a 'sentence finisher' for other people and has slowly learnt to focus attention on the other person and really listen to them.

7 COUNSELLING SKILLS II: CLIENT CENTRED SKILLS

Counselling skills may be divided into two subgroups: listening and attending, and counselling interventions. Listening and attending were considered in the last chapter. This chapter identifies important counselling interventions: the things that the counsellor says in the counselling relationship.

The term 'client centred', first used by Carl Rogers (1951), refers to the notion that the client himself is best able to decide how to find the solutions to his problems in living. 'Client centred', in this sense, may be contrasted with the idea of 'counsellor centred' or 'professional centred', both of which may suggest that someone other than the client is the 'expert'. Whilst this may be true when applied to certain concrete 'factual' problems – housing, surgery, legal problems and so forth – it is difficult to see how it can apply to personal life issues. In such cases, it is the client who identifies the problem and the client who, given time and space, can find their way through the problem to the solution.

Murgatroyd (1986) summarizes the client-centred position as follows.

- A person in need has come to you for help
- In order to be helped, they need to know that you have understood how they think and feel
- They also need to know that, whatever your own feelings about who or what they are or what they have or have not done, you accept them as they are.
- You accept their right to decide their own lives for themselves
- In the light of this knowledge about your acceptance and understanding of them they will begin to open themselves to the possibility of change and development.
- But if they feel that their association with you is conditional upon them changing, they may feel pressurized and reject your help.

The first issues identified by Murgatroyd, the fact of the client coming for help and needing to be understood and accepted, have been discussed in previous chapters. What we need to consider now are ways of helping the person to express themselves, to open themselves and thus to begin to change. It is worth noting, too, the almost paradoxical nature of Murgatroyd's last point: that if the client feels that their association with you is conditional upon them changing, they may reject your help. Thus we enter into the counselling relationship without even being desirous of the other person changing!

In a sense, this is an impossible state of affairs. If we did not hope for change, we presumably would not enter into the task of counselling in the first place. On another level, however, the point is a very important one. People change at their own rate and in their own time. The process cannot be rushed and we cannot will another person to change. Nor can we expect them to change to become more the sort of person that we would like them to be. We must meet them on their own terms and observe change as they wish and will it to be (or not, as the case may be). This sort of counselling, then, is very altruistic. It demands of us that we make no demands of others.

Client-centred counselling is a process rather than a particular set of skills. It evolves through the relationship that the counsellor has with the client and vice versa. In a sense, it is a period of growth for both parties, for each learns from the other. It also involves the exercise of restraint. The counsellor must restrain herself from offering advice and from the temptation to 'put the client's life right' for him. The outcome of such counselling cannot be predicted nor can concrete goals be set (unless they are devised by the client, at their request). In essence, client centred counselling involves an act of faith: a belief in the other person's ability to find solutions through the process of therapeutic conversation and through the act of being engaged in a close relationship with another human being.

Certain basic client centred skills may be identified although, as we have noted, it is the total relationship that is important. Skills exercised in isolation amount to little: the warmth, genuineness and positive regard must also be present. On the other hand, if basic skills are not considered, then the counselling process will probably be shapeless or it will degenerate into the counsellor becoming prescriptive. The skill of standing back and allowing the client to find his own way is a difficult one to learn. The following factors may help in the process:

- questions;
- reflection;
- selective reflection;
- empathy building;
- checking for understanding.

Each of these skills will now be considered in turn and in the last chapter a wide range of exercises is offered for the development of the skills. Each skill can be learned. In order for that to happen, each must be tried and practised. There is a temptation to say 'I do that anyway!' when reading a description of some of these skills. The point is to notice the doing of them and to practise doing them better!

Whilst counselling often shares the characteristics of everyday conversation, if it is to progress beyond that it is important that some, if not all, of the following skills are used effectively, tactfully and skilfully.

QUESTIONS

Two main sorts of questions may be identified in the client centred approach: closed and open questions. A closed question is one that elicits a 'yes', 'no' or similar one-word answer. Or it is one for which the counsellor can anticipate an approximation of the answer, as she asks it. Examples of closed questions are as follows.

- What is your name?
- How many children do you have?
- Are you happier now?
- Are you still depressed?

Too many closed questions can make the counselling relationship seem like an interrogation! They also inhibit the client in the telling of his story and place the locus of responsibility in the relationship firmly with the client. Consider, for instance, the following exchange between marriage guidance counsellor and client

Counsellor: Are you happier now . . . at home?
Client: Yes, I think I am...
Counsellor: Is that because you can talk more easily with your wife?
Client: I think so . . . we seem to get on better, generally.
Counsellor: And has your wife noticed the difference?
Client: Yes, she has.

In this exchange, made up only of closed questions, the counsellor clearly 'leads' the conversation. She also tends to try to influence the client towards accepting the idea that he is 'happier now' and that his wife has 'noticed the difference'. One of the problems with this sort of questioning is that it gives little opportunity for the client to profoundly disagree with the counsellor. In the above exchange, for example, could the client easily have disagreed with the counsellor? It would seem not.

On the other hand, the closed question is useful in clarifying certain specific issues. For example, one may be used as follows.

Client: It's not always easy at home . . . the children always seem to be so noisy . . . and my wife finds it difficult to cope with them . . .
Counsellor: How many children have you?
Client: Three. They're all under ten and they're at the sort of age when they use up a lot of energy and make a lot of noise . . .

Here, the closed question is fairly unobtrusive and serves to clarify the conversation. Notice, too, that once the question has been asked, the counsellor allows the client to continue to talk about his family, without further interruption.

Open questions

Open questions are those that do not elicit a particular answer: the counsellor cannot easily anticipate what an answer will 'look like'. Examples of open questions include the following.

- What did you do then?
- How did you feel when that happened?
- How are you feeling right now?
- What do you think will happen?

Open questions are ones that encourage the client to say more, to expand on their story or to go deeper. An example of their use is as follows.

Counsellor: What is happening at home at the moment?
Client: Things are going quite well. Everyone's much more settled now and my son's found himself a job. He's been out of work for a long time . . .
Counsellor: How have you felt about that?
Client: It's upset me a lot . . . It seemed wrong that I was working and he wasn't . . . he had to struggle for a long time . . . he wasn't happy at all . . .
Counsellor: And how are you feeling right now?
Client: Upset . . . I'm still upset . . . I still feel that I didn't help him enough . . .

In this conversation, the counsellor uses only open questions and the client expands on what he thinks and feels. More importantly, perhaps, the above example illustrates the counsellor 'following' the client and noting his paralinguistic and non-verbal cues. In this way, she is able to help the client to focus more on what is happening in the present. This is an example of the 'concreteness' and 'immediacy' referred to in Chapter 3.

Open questions are generally preferable, in counselling, to closed ones. They encourage longer, more expansive answers and are rather more free of value judgements and interpretation than are closed questions. All the same, the counsellor has to monitor the 'slope' of intervention when using open questions. It is easy, for example, to become intrusive by asking too piercing questions, too quickly. As with all counselling interventions, the timing of the use of questions is vital.

When to use questions

Questions can be used in counselling relationships for a variety of purposes. The main ones include the following.

- Exploration: 'What else happened...?', 'How did you feel then?'
- For further information: 'How many children have you got?', 'What sort of work were you doing before you retired?'
- To clarify: 'I'm sorry, did you say you are going to move or did you say you're not sure?', 'What did you say then. . . ?'
- Encouraging client to talk: 'Can you say more about that?', 'What are your feelings about that?'

Other sorts of questions

There are other ways of classifying questions and some to be avoided!

Leading questions

These are questions that contain an assumption which places the client in an untenable position. The classic example of a leading question is: 'Have you stopped beating your wife?'! Clearly, however the question is answered, the client is in the wrong! Other examples of leading questions are:

- Is your depression the thing that's making your work so difficult?
- Are your family upset by your behaviour?
- Do you think that you may be hiding something . . . even from yourself?

The last, pseudo analytical question is particularly awkward. What could the answer possibly be?

Value-laden questions

Questions such as 'Does your homosexuality make you feel guilty?' not only pose a moral question but guarantee that the client feels difficult answering it!

'Why' questions

These have been discussed in Chapter 3 and the problems caused by them in the counselling relationship suggest that they should be used very sparingly, if at all.

Confronting questions

Examples of these may include: 'Can you give me an example of when that happened?' and 'Do you still love your wife'. Confrontation in counselling is quite appropriate once the relationship has fully developed but needs to be used skilfully and appropriately. It is easy for apparent 'confrontation' to degenerate into moralizing. Heron (1986) and Schulman (1982) offer useful approaches to effective confrontation in counselling.

Funnelling

Funnelling (Kahn and Cannell, 1957) refers to the use of questions to guide the conversation from the general to the specific. Thus, the conversation starts with broad, opening questions and slowly, more specific questions are used to focus the discussion. An example of the use of funnelling follows.

Counsellor: You seem upset at the moment, what's happening?
Client: Its home . . . things aren't working out . . .
Counsellor: What's happening at home?
Client: I'm always falling out with Jane and the children . . .

Counsellor: What does Jane feel about what's happening?
Client: She's angry with me . . .
Counsellor: About something in particular?
Client: Yes, about the way I talk to Andrew, my son . . .
Counsellor: What is the problem with Andrew?

In this way, the conversation becomes directed and focused . . . and this may pose a problem. If the counsellor does use funnelling in this way, it is arguable that the counselling conversation is no longer client centred but counsellor directed. Perhaps, in many situations – particularly where shortage of time is an issue – a combination of following and leading may be appropriate. Following refers to the counsellor taking the lead from the client and exploring the avenues that he wants to explore. Leading refers to the counsellor taking a more active role and pursuing certain issues that she feels are important. If in doubt, however, the 'following' approach is probably preferable as it keeps the locus of control firmly with the client.

Funnelling in Practice

Andy is a volunteer telephone counsellor on a local AIDS Helpline. A young man of 18 rings in to ask about the symptoms of AIDS and for general information about the condition. Andy, in return, asks some open questions of the young man in order to establish a 'phone relationship'. As the conversation progresses, Andy gradually asks more specific questions and helps the young man to express more particular, personal anxieties about his own sexuality and his fear that he may be homosexual. Using the 'funnelling' approach, Andy is able to help the man through a difficult personal crisis that continues to be worked through in subsequent counselling sessions.

REFLECTION

Reflection (sometimes called 'echoing') is the process of reflecting back the last few words, or a paraphrase of the last few words, that the client has used, in order to encourage them to say more. It is as though the counsellor is echoing the client's thoughts and as though that echo serves as a prompt. It is important that the reflection does not turn into a question and this is best achieved by the counsellor making the repetition in much the same tone of voice as the client used. An example of the use of reflection is as follows.

Client: We had lived in the South for a number of years. Then we moved and I suppose that's when things started to go wrong . . .
Counsellor: Things started to go wrong . . .
Client: Well, we never really settled down. My wife missed her friends and I suppose I did really . . . though neither of us said anything . . .
Counsellor: Neither of you said that you missed your friends . . .
Client: We both tried to protect each other, really. I suppose if either of

us had said anything, we would have felt that we were letting the other one down . . .

In this example, the reflections are unobtrusive and unnoticed by the client. They serve to help the client to say more, to develop his story. Used skilfully and with good timing, reflection can be an important method of helping the client. On the other hand, if it is overused or used clumsily, it can appear stilted and is very noticeable. Unfortunately, it is an intervention that takes some practice and one that many people anticipate learning on counselling courses. As a result, when people return from counselling courses, their friends and relatives are often waiting for them to use the technique and may comment on the fact! This should not be a deterrent as the method remains a useful and therapeutic one.

Selective reflection

Selective reflection refers to the method of repeating back to the client a part of something they said that was emphasized in some way or which seemed to be emotionally charged. Thus selective reflection draws from the middle of the client's utterance and not from the end. An example of the use of selective reflection is as follows.

Client: We had just got married. I was very young and I thought things would work out OK. We started buying our own house. My wife hated the place! It was important, though . . . we had to start somewhere . . .

Counsellor: Your wife hated the house . . .

Client: She thought it was the worst place she'd lived in! She reckoned that she would only live there for a year at the most and we ended up being there for five years!

The use of selective reflection allowed the client in this example to develop further an almost throwaway remark. Often, these 'asides' are the substance of very important feelings and the counsellor can often help in their release by using selective reflection to focus on them. Clearly, concentration is important, in order to note the points on which to selectively reflect. Also, the counselling relationship is a flowing, evolving conversation which tends to be 'seamless'. Thus, the counsellor should not store up a point which she feels would be useful to selectively reflect! By the time a break comes in the conversation, the item will probably be irrelevant! This points up, again, the need to develop 'free-floating attention': the ability to allow the ebb and flow of the conversation to go where the client takes it and for the counsellor to trust her own ability to choose an appropriate intervention when a break occurs.

EMPATHY-BUILDING

This refers to the counsellor making statements to the client that indicate that she has understood the feeling the client is experiencing. A certain intuitive ability is needed here, for often empathy-building statements refer more to what is implied than what is overtly said. An example of the use of empathy building statements is as follows.

Client: People at work are the same. They're all tied up with their own friends and families . . . they don't have a lot of time for me . . . though they're friendly enough . . .
Counsellor: You sound angry with them . . .
Client: I suppose I am! Why don't they take a bit of time to ask me how I'm getting on? It wouldn't take much! . . .
Counsellor: It sounds as though you are saying that people haven't had time for you for a long time . . .
Client: They haven't. My family didn't bother much . . . I mean, they looked as though they did . . . but they didn't really . . .

Empathy-building statements read between the lines. Now, sometimes such reading can be completely wrong and the empathy-building statement is rejected by the client. When this happens, it is important for the counsellor to drop the approach altogether and to pay more attention to listening. Inaccurate empathy-building statements often indicate an overwillingness on the part of the counsellor to become 'involved' with the client's perceptual world – at the expense of accurate empathy! Used skilfully, however, they help the client to disclose further and indicate to the client that they are understood.

CHECKING FOR UNDERSTANDING

Checking for understanding involves either (a) asking the client if you have understood them correctly or (b) occasionally summarizing the conversation in order to clarify what has been said. The first type of checking is useful when the client quickly covers a lot of topics and seems to be 'thinking aloud'. It can be used to further focus the conversation or as a means of ensuring that the counsellor really stays with what the client is saying. The second type of checking should be used sparingly or the counselling conversation can get to seem rather mechanical and studied. The following two examples illustrate the two uses of checking for understanding.

Example 1
Client: I feel all over the place at the moment . . . things aren't quite right at work . . . money is still a problem and I don't seem to be talking to anyone . . . I'm not sure about work . . . sometimes I feel like packing it in . . . at other times I think I'm doing OK . . .
Counsellor: Let me just clarify . . . you're saying things are generally a problem at the moment and you've thought about leaving work?
Client: Yes . . . I don't think I will stop work but if I can get to talk it over with my boss, I think I will feel easier about it.

Example 2
Counsellor: Let me see if I can just sum up what we've talked about this afternoon. We talked about the financial problems and the question of talking to the bank manager. You suggested that you may ask him for a loan. Then you went on to say how you felt you could organize your finances better in the future. . . ?
Client: Yes, I think that covers most things . . .

Some counsellors prefer to use the second type of checking at the end of each counselling session and this may help to clarify things before the client leaves. On the other hand, there is much to be said for not 'tidying up' the end of the session in this way. If the loose ends are left, the client continues to think about all the issues that have been discussed as he walks away from the session. If everything is summarized too neatly, the client may feel that the problems can be 'closed down' for a while or, even worse, that they have been 'solved'! Personal problems are rarely simple enough to be summarized in a few words and checking at the end of a session should be used sparingly.

These, then, are particular skills that encourage self-direction on the part of the client and can be learned and used by the counsellor. They form the basis of all good counselling and can always be returned to as a primary way of working with the client in the counselling relationship.

IS THE CLIENT CENTRED APPROACH ENOUGH?

The 1990s have seen many changes in health provision. They have also seen dramatic changes in people's financial, work and life situations. These changes have contributed to a considerable debate about the appropriateness of the client centred approach to counselling as an *exclusive* approach. Writing of the development of humanistic psychology in counselling, Dryden *et al.* (1989) have this to say:

> ***The object of person-centred counselling . . . is to help the client 'to become what he/she is capable of becoming' (Rogers 1951), or, to employ an even more well-worn phrase associated with Maslow, to achieve self-actualization (Maslow 1962). These terms have a slightly hollow ring about them in the enterprise economy of the late 1980s in Britain, in which the division between the 'haves' and the 'have nots' is sharply apparent. Striving for self-actualization is easier if one is well-off, well-housed, has a rewarding and secure job and lives in a pleasant environment than if one is unemployed, poor, ill-housed, and lives in a run-down neighbourhood. Terms like self-actualization simply do not feature in and do not derive from the culture of the 1980s.***

Howard (1990) made a similar point rather more directly when, discussing the changing needs of clients who seek counselling, he suggested about counsellors that:

> *It is time we shed our naivety and the 'syrupy' illusions of Carl Rogers and his many cohorts.*

These writers raise important questions that relate to issues in this study. There have been considerable changes in life in the UK since the 1960s. The political climate has changed, employment patterns and patterns of health and sickness have also changed, some would say irreversibly (Bowen, 1990). Ashton and Seymour (1988) sum up some of these changes as follows.

> *Fundamental changes are taking place both in the way we view ill-health and the way individuals, families and governments respond to it. In the United Kingdom ministerial reputations and careers are being made and lost out of the health-related issues of AIDS, drugs, heart disease and the environmental conditions of the inner cities. The once sacred National Health Service is under attack for failing to deliver the goods and the long assumed immunity to accountability of physicians is falling away week by week. In Liverpool, 26 per cent of adult men are unemployed and nationally the infant mortality rate has just risen for the first time in 16 years.*

Ashton and Seymour begin to raise the question of whether or not the client centred approach is appropriate in AIDS counselling. In the next chapter, it is noted that education and advice both have their part to play in effective AIDS counselling. It is also noted that the concept of AIDS counselling involves a wide and diverse range of counselling. Thus, it seems likely that a more *prescriptive* approach to counselling may be appropriate in the AIDS field. On the other hand, Rogers was not only advocating a particular set of skills or counselling interventions, he was also suggesting a particular *attitude* towards counselling which involved respect for the client, appreciation of their range of choices and the fact that it was the client who, in the end, made their decision for themselves. This aspect of the Rogerian approach may still be appropriate in all types of counselling.

Murgatroyd and Woolfe (1982) note that approaches to counselling and caring for people with different problems of living are also changing. They suggest that there has been a move away from the client centred approach of Rogers towards an interest in short-term, crisis-oriented counselling for which more directive, action-oriented procedures are usually advocated.

A number of commentators and researchers have also moved away from the client centred approach to counselling towards a more challenging one and see confrontation and challenge as an essential part of the counselling process (Dorn, 1986; Ellis, 1987; Ellis and Dryden, 1987). Farrelly and Brandsma (1974) propose four 'challenge-related hypotheses' for consideration within the counselling movement.

1 Clients can change if they choose.
2 Clients have more resources for managing problems in living and developing opportunities than they or most helpers assume.
3 The psychological fragility of clients is over-rated by both themselves and others.
4 Maladaptive and antisocial attitudes and behaviours of clients can be significantly altered no matter what the degree of severity or chronicity.

In a similar vein, Howard *et al.*, (1987) suggest that action and challenge are an essential part of human make-up and that people have a 'bias towards action' which requires them, directly or indirectly, to:

- change from a passive to a more active state;
- change from a state of dependency on others to relative independence;
- change from behaving in a few ways to acting in many ways;
- change in interests – with erratic, shallow and casual interests giving way to mature, strong and enduring interests;
- change from a present-oriented time perspective to a perspective encompassing past, present and future;
- change from solely subordinate relationships with others to relationship as equals or superiors;
- change from lack of a clear sense of self to a clearer sense of self and control of self.

As with most things, there needs to be a middle path. Sometimes, the client centred approach will suffice. At other times, a more confronting approach may be appropriate. Also, there are situations in which the giving of clear information is important. In Chapter 9, some of these situations are explored in greater detail. The most obvious current situation is that of people who, for whatever reason, find themselves in the HIV/AIDS field.

Despite criticisms and limitations, the client-centred approach continues to be useful and practical in a variety of health care settings. As Davis and Fallowfield (1991) suggest:

> ***Rogers presented his theories as a basis for development, and not as complete and absolute frameworks. He was at pains to express his ideas tentatively and clearly, pointing out what was unknown or less than certain.***

However, we are likely to see changes. The client-centred approach may be time consuming and it is difficult to evaluate for effectiveness. As we have noted elsewhere, health care in the UK and other countries is changing. The push towards *evidence-based practice* is everywhere and counsellors, like all other practitioners, have to be able to demonstrate how well or otherwise their practice 'works'.

The client centred approach in practice

Mary, a health visitor, is asked by one of her young single-parent clients about her young daughter's inability to sleep. Mary uses client centred interventions and draws out the details surrounding the family situation. In encouraging the young mother to talk through her financial and emotional worries, she allows some of the pressure on the mother to be dispelled. She follows this up with some practical suggestions about how to help the daughter to sleep, including the suggestions of a regular bedtime, a planned routine during the evening and a 'winding down' period before going to bed. The combination of allowing the mother to talk out her own anxieties and offering practical suggestions enables both mother and daughter to live more comfortably.

CLIENT CENTRED SKILLS AND THE HEALTH PROFESSIONAL

Whilst the discussion in this chapter has focused on the use of client-centred interventions in the counselling relationship, the range of skills involved is clearly useful in a wide range of health contexts. Workers in the primary health care team may use them as part of their assessment programme whilst professionals in longer term care can use them as supportive measures and as a means of evaluating the effectiveness of care. In nursing, they may be used to draw up care plans and to implement, effectively, the use of nursing models – particularly self-care models. In the next chapter, we will look at how to combine these client centred interventions with those that help clients to express and handle emotions and feelings.

8 Counselling skills III: helping with feelings

A considerable part of the process of helping people in counselling is concerned with the emotional or 'feelings' side of the person. In British and North American cultures, a great premium is placed on the individual's being able to 'control' feelings and thus overt expression of emotion is often frowned upon. As a result, we learn to bottle up feelings, sometimes from a very early age. Dorothy Rowe (1987) has summed up the situation well.

> ***Just as we were born with the ability to breathe so we were born with the ability to express our emotions fully and to be aware of other people's emotions. We can keep our capacity to experience the full range and totality of our feelings and our capacity to empathize with other people. We can use these capacities to know ourselves, to know other people and let them be themselves. We can do this. But we rarely do. Society, the group we belong to, will not let us.***

In this chapter, we will consider the effects of such suppression of feelings and identify some practical ways of helping people to identify and explore their feelings. The skills involved in managing feelings can be seen to augment the skills discussed in the previous chapter – the basic client centred counselling skills.

Types of emotion

Heron (1977a) distinguishes between at least four types of emotion that are commonly suppressed or bottled up: anger, fear, grief and embarrassment. He notes a relationship between these feelings and certain overt expressions of them. Thus, in counselling, anger may be expressed as loud sound, fear as trembling, grief through tears and embarrassment by laughter. He notes, also, a relationship between those feelings and certain basic human needs. Heron argues that we all need to understand and know what is happening to us. If that knowledge is not forthcoming, we may experience fear. We need, also, to make choices in our lives and if that choice is restricted in certain ways, we may feel anger. Third, we need to experience the expression of love and of being loved. If that love is denied us or taken away from us, we may experience grief. To Heron's basic human needs may be added the need for self-respect and dignity. If such dignity is denied us, we may feel self-conscious and embarrassed. Practical examples of how these relationships 'work' in everyday life and in the counselling relationship may be illustrated as follows.

A 20-year-old girl is attempting to live in a flat on her own. Her parents, however, insist on visiting her regularly and making suggestions as to how she should decorate the flat. They also regularly buy her articles for it and gradually she senses that she is feeling very uncomfortable and distanced from her parents. In the counselling relationship she discovers that she is very angry: her desire to make choices for herself is continually being eroded by her parents' benevolence.

A 45-year-old man hears that his mother is seriously ill and subsequently she dies. He feels no emotions except that of feeling 'frozen' and unemotional. During a counselling session he suddenly discovers the need to cry profoundly. As he does so, he realizes that, many years ago, he had decided that crying was not a masculine thing to do. As a result, he blocked off his grief and felt numb until, within the safety of the counselling relationship, he was able to discover his grief and express it.

An 18-year-old boy, discussing his college work during a counselling session, begins to laugh almost uncontrollably. As he does so, he begins to feel the laughter turning to tears. Through his mixed laughter and tears he acknowledges that 'No-one ever took me seriously . . . not at school, at home . . . or anywhere'. His laughter may be an expression of his lack of self-esteem and his tears, the grief he experiences at that lack.

In the last example it may be noted how emotions that are suppressed are rarely only of one sort. Very often, bottled-up emotion is a mixture of anger, fear, embarrassment and grief. Often, too, the causes of such blocked emotion are unclear and lost in the history of the person. It is perhaps more important that the expression of pent-up emotion is often helpful in that it seems to allow the person to be clearer in his thinking once he has expressed it. It is as though the blocked emotion 'gets in the way' and its release acts as a means of helping the person to clarify his thoughts and feelings. It is notable that the suppression of feelings can lead to certain problems in living that may be clearly identified.

THE EFFECTS OF BOTTLING UP EMOTION

Physical discomfort and muscular pain

Wilhelm Reich, a psychoanalyst with a particular interest in the relationship between emotions and the musculature, noted that blocked emotions could become trapped in the body's muscle clusters (Reich, 1949). He noted that anger was frequently 'trapped' in the muscles of the shoulders, grief in muscles surrounding the stomach and fear in the leg muscles. Often, these trapped emotions lead to chronic postural problems. Sometimes, the thorough release of the blocked emotion can lead to a freeing up of the muscles and an improved physical appearance. Reich believed in working directly on the muscle clusters in order to bring about emotional release and subsequent freedom from suppression and out of his work was developed a particular type of mind/body therapy, known as 'bioenergetics' (Lowen, 1967; Lowen and Lowen, 1977).

In terms of everyday counselling, trapped emotion is sometimes 'visible' in the way that the client holds himself and the skilled counsellor can learn to notice tension in the musculature and changes in breathing patterns that may suggest muscular tension. We have noted throughout this book how difficult it is to interpret another person's behaviour. What is important here is that such bodily manifestations be used only as a clue to what may be happening in the person. We cannot assume that a person who looks tense, is tense until he has said that he is.

Health professionals will be very familiar with the link between body posture, the musculature and the emotional state of the person. Frequently, if patients and clients can be helped to relax, then their medical and psychological condition may improve more quickly. Those health professionals who deal most directly with the muscle clusters (remedial gymnasts and physiotherapists, for example) will tend to notice physical tension more readily but all carers can train themselves to observe these important indicators of the emotional status of the person in their care.

Difficulty in decision making

This is a frequent side-effect of bottled-up emotion. It is as though the emotion makes the person uneasy and that uneasiness leads to lack of confidence. As a result, that person finds it difficult to rely on his own resources and may find decision making difficult. When we are under stress of any sort, we often feel the need to check decisions with other people. Once some of this stress is removed by talking through problems or by releasing pent-up emotions, the decision-making process often becomes easier.

Faulty self-image

When we bottle up feelings, those feelings often have an unpleasant habit of turning against us. Thus, instead of expressing anger towards others, we turn it against ourselves and feel depressed as a result. Or, if we have hung onto unexpressed grief, we turn that grief in on ourselves and experience ourselves as less than we are. Often, in counselling, as old resentments or dissatisfactions are expressed, so the person begins to feel better about himself.

Setting unrealistic goals

Tension can lead to further tension. This tension can lead us to set ourselves unreachable targets. It is almost as though we set ourselves up to fail! Sometimes, too, failing is a way of punishing ourselves or it is 'safer' than achieving. Release of tension, through the expression of emotion, can sometimes help a person to take a more realistic view of himself and his goal setting.

The development of long-term faulty beliefs

Sometimes, emotion that has been bottled up for a long time can lead to a person's view of the world being coloured in a particular way. He learns that 'people can't be trusted' or 'people always let you down in the end'. It is as though old, painful feelings lead to distortions that become part of that person's worldview. Such long-term distorted beliefs about the world do not change easily but may be modified as the person comes to release feelings and learns to handle his emotions more effectively.

The 'last straw' syndrome

Sometimes, if emotion is bottled up for a considerable amount of time, a valve blows and the person hits out – either literally or verbally. We have all experienced the problem of storing up anger and taking it out on someone else, a process that is sometimes called 'displacement'. The original object of our anger is now replaced by something or someone else. Again, the talking through of difficulties or the release of pent-up emotion can often help to ensure that the person does not feel the need to explode in this way.

Clearly, no two people react to the bottling up of emotion in the same way. Some people, too, choose not to deal with life events emotionally. It would be curious to argue that there is a 'norm' where emotions are concerned. On the other hand, many people complain of being unable to cope with emotions and if the client perceives there to be a problem in the emotional domain, then that perception may be expressed as a desire to explore his emotional status. It is important, however, that the counsellor does not force her particular set of beliefs about feelings and emotions on the client, but waits to be asked to help. Often the request for such help is tacit: the client talks about difficulty in dealing with emotion and that, in itself, may safely be taken as a request for help. A variety of methods is available to the counsellor to help in the exploration of the domain of feelings and those methods will be described. Sometimes, these methods produce catharsis: the expression of strong emotion – tears, anger, fear, laughter. Drawing on the literature on the subject, the following statements may be made about the handling of such emotional release.

- Emotional release is usually self-limiting. If the person is allowed to cry or get angry, that emotion will be expressed and then gradually subside. The supportive counsellor will allow it to happen and not become unduly distressed by it.
- Physical support can sometimes be helpful in the form of holding the person's hand or putting an arm round them. Care should be taken, however, that such actions are unambiguous and that the holding of the client is not too 'tight'. A very tight embrace is likely to inhibit the release of emotion. It is worth remembering, also, that not everyone likes or wants physical contact. It is important the counsellor's support is not seen as intrusive by the client.
- Once the person has had a cathartic release they will need time to piece together the insights that they gain from it. Often, all that is needed is that the counsellor sits quietly with the client while he occasionally verbalizes what he is thinking. The postcathartic period can be a very important stage in the counselling process.
- There seems to be a link between the extent to which we can

'allow' another person to express emotion and the degree to which we can handle our own emotion. This is another reason why the counsellor needs self-awareness. To help others explore their feelings we need, first, to explore our own. Many colleges and university departments offer workshops on cathartic work and self-awareness development that can help both in training the counsellor to help others and in gaining self-insight.

- Frequent 'cathartic counselling' can be exhausting for the counsellor and if she is to avoid burnout, she needs to set up a network of support from other colleagues or via a peer support group. We cannot hope to constantly handle other people's emotional release without its taking a toll on us.

METHODS OF HELPING THE CLIENT TO EXPLORE FEELINGS

These are practical methods that can be used in the counselling relationship to help the client to identify, examine and, if required, release emotion. Most of them will be more effective if the counsellor has first tried them on herself. This can be done simply by reading through the description of them and then trying them out, in your mind. Alternatively, they can be tried out with a colleague or friend. Another way of exploring their effectiveness is to use them in a peer support context. The setting up and running of such a group is described in the final chapter of this book, along with various exercises that can be used to improve counselling skills. All the following activities should be used gently and thoughtfully and timed to fit in with the client's requirements. There should never be any sense of pushing the client to explore feelings because of a misplaced belief that 'a good cry will do him good!'.

Giving permission

Sometimes in counselling, the client tries desperately to hang on to strong feelings and not to express them. As we have seen, this may be due to the cultural norm which suggests that holding on is often better than letting go. Thus a primary method for helping someone to explore his emotions is for the counsellor to 'give permission' for the expression of feeling. This can be done simply through acknowledging that 'It's all right with me if you feel you are going to cry . . .' In this way the counsellor has reassured the client that expression of feelings is acceptable within the relationship. Clearly, a degree of tact is required here. It is important that the client does not feel pushed into expressing feelings that he would rather not express. The 'permission giving' should never be coercive nor should there be an implicit suggestion that 'you must express your feelings!'.

Literal description

This refers to inviting the client to go back in his memory to a place that he has, until now, only alluded to and describe that place in some detail. An example of this use of literal description is as follows.

Client: I used to get like this at home . . . I used to get very upset . . .
Counsellor: Just go back home for a moment . . . describe one of the rooms in the house . . .
Client: The front room faces directly out onto the street . . . there is an armchair by the window . . . the TV in the corner . . . our dog is lying on the rug . . . it's very quiet . . .
Counsellor: What are you feeling right now?
Client: Like I was then . . . angry . . . upset . . .

Describing in literal terms a place that was the scene of an emotional experience can often bring that emotion back. When the counsellor has invited the client to literally describe a particular place, she then asks him to identify the feeling that emerges from that description. It is important that the description has an 'I am there' quality about it and does not slip into a detached description, such as: 'We lived in a big house which wasn't particularly modern but then my parents didn't like modern houses much . . .'

Locating and developing a feeling in terms of the body

As we have noted above, very often feelings are accompanied by a physical sensation. It is often helpful to identify that physical experience and to invite the client to exaggerate it, to allow the feeling to 'expand' in order to explore it further. An example of this approach is as follows.

Counsellor: How are you feeling at the moment?
Client: Slightly anxious.
Counsellor: Where, in terms of your body, do you feel the anxiety?
Client: (rubs stomach) Here
Counsellor: Can you increase that feeling in your stomach?
Client: Yes, it's spreading up to my chest.
Counsellor: And what's happening now?
Client: It reminds me of a long time ago . . . when I first started work . . .
Counsellor What happened there. . . ?

Again, the original suggestion by the counsellor is followed through by a question to elicit how the client is feeling following the suggestion. This gives the client a chance to identify the thoughts that go with the feeling and to explore them further.

Empty chair

Another method of exploring feelings is to invite the client to imagine the feeling that they are experiencing as 'sitting' in a chair next to them and then have them address the feeling. This can be used in a variety of ways and the next examples show its applications.

Example 1
Client: I feel very confused at the moment, I can't seem to sort things out . . .

Counsellor: Can you imagine your confusion sitting in that chair over there . . . what does it look like?
Client: It looks like a great big ball of wool . . . how odd!
Counsellor: If you could speak to your confusion, what would you say to it?
Client: I wish I could sort you out!
Counsellor: And what's your confusion saying back to you?
Client: I'm glad you don't sort me out – I stop you from having to make any decisions!
Counsellor: And what do you make of that?
Client: I suppose that could be true . . . the longer I stay confused, the less I have to make decisions about my family . . . .

Example 2
Counsellor: How are you feeling about the people you work with . . . you said you found it quite difficult to get on with them . . .
Client: Yes, it's still difficult, especially my boss.
Counsellor: Imagine your boss is sitting in that chair over there . . . how does that feel?
Client: Uncomfortable! He's angry with me!
Counsellor: What would you like to say to him?
Client: Why do I always feel scared of you . . . why do you make me feel uncomfortable?
Counsellor: And what does he say?
Client: I don't! It's you that feels uncomfortable, not me . . . You make yourself uncomfortable . . . (to the counsellor) He's right! I do make myself uncomfortable but I use him as an excuse . . .

The 'empty chair' can be used in a variety of ways to set up a dialogue between either the client and his feelings or the client and a person that the client talks 'about'. It offers a very direct way of exploring relationships and feelings and deals directly with the issue of 'projection' – the tendency we have to see qualities in others that are, in fact, our own. Using the 'empty chair' technique can bring to light those projections and allow the client to see them for what they are. Other applications of this method are described in detail by Perls (1969).

Contradiction

It is sometimes helpful if the client is asked to contradict a statement that they make, especially when that statement contains some ambiguity. An example of this approach is as follows.

Client: (looking at the floor) I've sorted everything out now: everything's OK.
Counsellor: Try contradicting what you've just said . . .
Client: Everything's not OK . . . Everything isn't sorted out . . . (laughs) . . . that's true, of course . . . there's a lot more to sort out yet . . .

Mobilization of body energy

Developing the idea discussed above that emotions can be trapped within the body's musculature, it is sometimes helpful for the counsellor to suggest to the client that he stretches or takes some very deep breaths. In the process, the client may become aware of tensions that are trapped in his body and begin to recognize and identify those tensions. This in turn can lead to the client talking about and expressing some of those tensions. This is particularly helpful if, during the counselling conversation, the client becomes less and less 'mobile' and adopts a particularly hunched or curled-up position in his chair. The invitation to stretch serves almost as a contradiction to the body position being adopted by the client at that time.

Exploring fantasy

We often set fairly arbitrary limits on what we think we can and cannot do. When a client seems to be doing this, it is sometimes helpful to explore what may happen if this limit was broken. An example of this is as follows.

Client: I'd like to be able to go abroad for a change, I never seem to go very far on holiday.
Counsellor: What stops you?
Client: Flying, I suppose . . .
Counsellor: What's the worst thing about flying?
Client: I get very anxious?
Counsellor: And what happens if you get very anxious?
Client: Nothing really! I just get anxious!
Counsellor: So nothing terrible will happen if you allow yourself to get anxious?
Client: No, not really . . . I hadn't thought about it like that before . . .

Rehearsal

Sometimes the anticipation of a coming event or situation provokes anxiety. The counsellor can usefully help the client to explore a range of feelings by rehearsing with him a future event. Thus the client who is anticipating a forthcoming interview may be helped by having the counsellor act the role of an interviewer, with a subsequent discussion. The client who wants to develop the assertive behaviour to enable him to challenge his boss may benefit from role playing the situation in the counselling session. In each case, it is important that both client and counsellor 'get into role' and that the session does not just become a discussion of what may or may not happen. The actual playing through and rehearsal of a situation is nearly always more powerful than a discussion of it. Alberti and Emmons (1982) offer some useful suggestions about how to set up role plays and exercises for developing assertive behaviour and Wilkinson and Canter (1982) describe some useful approaches to developing socially skilled behaviour. Often, if the client can practise effective behaviour, then the appropriate thoughts and feelings can accompany that behaviour. The novelist Kurt Vonnegut wryly commented that: 'We are what we pretend to be – so take care what you pretend to be' (Vonnegut, 1968). Sometimes, the first stage in changing is trying out a new pattern of behaviour or a new way of thinking and feeling. Practice, therefore, is invaluable.

This approach develops from the idea that what we think influences what we feel and do. If our thinking is restrictive, we may begin to feel that we can or cannot do certain things. Sometimes, having these barriers to feeling and doing challenged can free a person to think, feel and act differently.

These methods of exploring feelings can be used alongside the client-centred interventions described in the previous chapter. They need to be practised so that the counsellor feels confident in using them; the means to developing the skills involved are identified in the final chapter of this book. The domain of feelings is one that is frequently addressed in counselling.

Counselling people who want to explore feelings takes time and cannot be rushed. Also, the development and use of the various skills described here is not the whole of the issue. Health professionals working with emotions also need to have developed the personal qualities described elsewhere: warmth, genuineness, empathic understanding and unconditional positive regard. Emotional counselling can never be a mechanical process but is one that touches the lives of both client and counsellor.

Helping with feelings in practice: I

Jane is a student nurse on a busy medical ward. She develops a close relationship with Arthur Davis, an elderly man who has been treated for heart failure. Suddenly and unexpectedly, Mr Davis dies. Jane finds herself unable to come to terms with this and seeks the help of an older tutor in the School of Nursing. The tutor helps her to talk through her feelings and she cries a great deal. Through the process of talking and crying she comes to realize that Arthur Davis reminded her of her own father, who had also died suddenly and for whom she had been unable to grieve. In grieving for Mr Davis, she was enabled to work through some of her grief for her own father.

Helping with feelings in practice: II

Andrew is a radiographer in a large casualty department. He has recently had difficulties in his marriage which he feels affect his work in the department. He is able to talk this through with his superintendent, who has had training as a counsellor. During the course of the conversation, Andrew feels close to tears. His superintendent says: 'What would happen if you allowed yourself to cry?'. Andrew smiles wryly and says 'nothing'. With that, he bursts into tears and is 'allowed' to cry. Afterwards, he finds it much easier to talk through his problems in a rational and systematic way and feels able to make more sense of what is happening at home. The superintendent's skilful and well-timed intervention gives Andrew the prompt that he needed to enable him to express bottled-up feelings.

HELPING WITH FEELINGS AND THE HEALTH PROFESSIONAL

As with other counselling interventions, those that deal with the expression of feelings have a wider application than just the counselling relationship. There are many occasions in health care when the professional is called upon to help and support the person who is in emotional distress. Sometimes, such situations arise as something of an emergency or arise suddenly and without warning. The professional who has considered the skills involved in helping with the expression of emotion will be better equipped to deal with these emergencies when they arise.

9 INFORMATION GIVING AND COUNSELLING IN SPECIFIC HEALTH CARE CONTEXTS

The climate of health care and the way in which people organize and live their lives are changing. As we have seen, there have been criticisms of the client centred approach to counselling. There are also situations in which giving clear and unequivocal advice is likely to be appropriate in counselling. In this chapter, three things are considered: information giving, counselling people in the HIV/AIDS field and talking to children. All three are current and important aspects of the counselling field in the health care professions.

INFORMATION GIVING

First, an important distinction needs to be made between *information giving* and *advice giving*. Information giving involves sharing with others facts, theories, statistics and other information gleaned from a variety of sources. Advice giving, on the other hand, suggests opinion: the *counsellor's* opinion. Whilst I have no intention of getting into the thorny debate about whether or not information can ever be 'objective' nor whether or not it can be proved to be 'true', there seems little doubt that information giving rarely involves a *moral* or *ethical* judgement that advice giving implies.

So far, this book has focused mostly on the client being 'drawn out' by the counsellor and on that client finding their way through problems to solutions. There are occasions, however, when those in a counselling role will be asked for specific information. This is true in all types of counselling but particularly in health care settings where the counsellor in question may have valuable and useful information to be shared with the client. Examples of situations in which information is required would include:

- the person who needs information about contraception;
- the person who is a newly diagnosed diabetic;
- the person who has recently been discharged from psychiatric hospital after many years;
- the person who is considering a career change but is unaware of options.

In all these situations, the counsellor is called upon to give information. If he or she does not have that information, then there is little point in bluffing or in trying to help the client to find it. In most cases it is more economical and safer to refer the person to another agency.

Certain guidelines can be offered about information giving. Information given in counselling should be:

- accurate;
- up to date;
- appropriate to the context;
- worded in such a way that the client will understand it;
- sufficient to satisfy the client's needs at the time.

Many health care professionals use jargon as a form of shorthand and as a means of quickly communicating with other colleagues. It is not difficult for such professionals to forget that they have learned this jargon and to assume that it is common currency amongst other people. It is vital that any health professional giving information does so using words that are straightforward, unambiguous and clear. This never means 'talking down' to the client but it does mean that that the counsellor should check with the client that they have understood the information that has been given. It is not uncommon for people to 'hear what they want to hear' – particularly when they are frightened or want to hear good news. Others are bemused by professionals and are uncertain how to seek clarification. The good counsellor will make themselves approachable enough to be questioned – at length, if necessary – by the client. Many of these points have been summarized, in the context of medicine, by Myerscough (1989).

> ***In addition to availability of information, a further element contributes greatly to the success of the exposition. This is the doctor's skill in choosing vocabulary suitable to the patient. The form of words and choice of terms will differ from one patient to another; it will be influenced by their education, cultural and occupational background and other factors. Terms the doctor may regard as 'innocent' and reassuring may readily create serious anxiety. For example, when a woman with a cervical erosion is told that she has 'just a small ulcer on the neck of the womb', she may infer the presence of serious disease, imminently or actually malignant, and be too alarmed to try to clarify what the doctor's words really mean.***

HIV/AIDS COUNSELLING: SOME CONSIDERATIONS

This section considers some of the issues that may concern the health professional as AIDS counsellor. It is important to state from the outset that just as not all health care professionals will need to develop counselling skills in general, nor will all health care professionals need to develop AIDS counselling skills.

It is possible to argue that the skills involved in counselling the person with AIDS are not fundamentally different from counselling anyone. On the other hand, the evidence suggests that people with AIDS often have particular problems that can best be helped by someone who has specific skills and knowledge (MacCaffrey, 1987; Andersen and MacElveen-Hoen, 1988; Sketchley, 1989).

Health care professionals are becoming increasingly interested in the issue of counselling as part of the nursing role (Hopper *et al.*, 1991; Tschudin, 1991). Also, it is clear from the developing literature on the topic that AIDS and AIDS counselling are issues of growing concern to health care professionals and educators in the UK (see, for example, Howe, 1989; Hurtig and Fandrick, 1990; McGough, 1990; Dennis, 1991).

Client groups

People who need AIDS counselling are not a homogeneous group. A list of the people who are likely to require counselling in this field is offered by Bor (1991):

- clients who have concerns or queries about AIDS, regardless of their clinical status;
- clients who are referred for the HIV antibody test;
- clients who are HIV antibody negative but who continue to present with AIDS-related worries;
- clients who are HIV antibody positive and symptomless;
- clients who are HIV antibody positive and who are becoming unwell;
- clients who have developed AIDS;
- clients who are being offered, or who are being considered for, antiviral treatments;
- the sexual contacts, loved ones or family of any of the above, if the client has given his or her permission;
- the close contacts of a deceased client, who may also later require bereavement counselling;
- staff with concerns about AIDS or those who are occupationally exposed to HIV (in conjunction with the occupational health department).

It seems clear that different sorts of counselling skills and approaches are likely to be needed in AIDS counselling and that 'AIDS counselling' is not one particular entity. Bor (1991) concludes that 'there are many different counselling approaches and no evidence yet that one is better than another'.

For people who are substance abusers, Cook *et al.* (1988) suggest risk reduction counselling, which includes:

1. assisting the client to acknowledge the personal risks of HIV infection;
2. explaining the range of changes that will reduce infection and transmission risks, addressing attitudinal and environmental obstacles (for example, feelings of having no control, resistance from partners) and rehearsing behaviours as needed;
3. reinforcing changes in a way that helps the client to assume increasing control over health behaviours so that early accomplishments can be sustained and built upon.

Faltz (1989) offers the following guidelines for working with substance-abusing clients, some of which may be appropriate for other client groups.

- Be willing to listen and encourage constructive expression of feelings;
- express caring and concern for the individual;
- hold the individual responsible for their actions;
- ensure consistent consequences for negative behaviours;
- talk to the individual about specific actions that are disruptive or disturbing;
- do not compromise your own values or expectations;
- communicate your plan of action to other staff members or professionals working with the client;
- monitor your own reactions to the client.

Many other sorts of clients have been discussed in the AIDS counselling literature, including 'the worried well', discussed in a little more detail below (Bor *et al.*, 1989); those who want or need to keep their diagnosis secret; the counselling of antenatal women (Miller and Bor, 1990); children (Miller *et al.*, 1989); those with haemophilia (DiMarzo, 1989); and ethnic minorities (Fullilove, 1989). Another group that might ask for counselling are bisexual people. The Off Pink Collective (1988), having noted the paucity of research into bisexuality, write as follows.

> ***Up until now the fact that maybe over a third of the population has strong attractions to or sexual activities with both sexes has generally been ignored. Sexual self-identities have been seen as either heterosexual, or gay or lesbian. But in reality people are not in distinct groups. As far as disease transmission is concerned, it is actual behaviour rather than self-identity that counts and many self-identified heterosexuals and gay men and lesbians behave bisexually. Contrary to a frequent association of bisexuality with promiscuity, it is our experience that many self-identified bisexuals are recurrently celibate and increasingly so as part of a safer sex life.***

Reviewing the literature on AIDS, AIDS counselling and sexuality tends to confirm the view that whilst bisexual people are noted to be at risk, they are less widely written about than are gay or heterosexual people.

There are specific issues in counselling for the counsellor who faces a person who is unsure about whether or not to be tested. McCreaner (1989) identifies the aims of pretest counselling as follows.

- To ensure that any decision to take the test is fully informed and based on an understanding of the personal, medical, legal and social implications of a positive result. At one level, this is a mere practical application of the traditional medical ethic of informed consent to a procedure.

- To provide the necessary preparation for those who will have to face the trauma of a positive result. Such preparation is vital in that patients who have been prepared for a positive result are able to face that result much more equably.
- To provide the individual, whether he eventually elects not to be tested, or elects to be tested and is found positive or found to be negative, with necessary risk reduction information on the basis of which he can reduce the risk of either acquiring HIV infection or passing it on to others.

For the person who has AIDS, Sketchley (1989) suggests that there are frequently four stages to be worked through in the counselling relationship:

- *Crisis*: a stage in which the predominant emotions are shock, fear and denial.
- *Adjustment to the news*: in which social disruption and withdrawal are common as the person struggles to accept the diagnosis.
- *Acceptance*: a stage in which the person adopts a new sense of self within the limitations imposed by the illness.
- *Preparation for death*: a stage in which the issues of fear of dependence, pain, being abandoned, isolation and death, itself, may predominate.

These stages are similar to those worked through by any person who has to face the prospect of dying (Stedeford, 1989). The counsellor who seeks to help the person with AIDS may also have to work on their feelings about their own death.

AIDS counselling is carried out by many people. At one level, various telephone counselling services exist for people who are worried that they may have AIDS and for those who need support. At another level, there are people who are identified specifically as AIDS counsellors (Leukefeld, 1988). They are often attached to hospitals, hospices and national AIDS organizations and offer help to people with AIDS, their friends and families (Dilley *et al.*,1989).

Different cities have organized their counselling and support systems in different ways. In 1987, the Canadian Federal Centre for AIDS observed that the AIDS programme in San Francisco was much more community oriented (with correspondingly more counselling agencies) than was the programme in New York (where many more people were being cared for in hospital).

Increasingly, health care professionals will find themselves fulfilling the role of AIDS counsellor for, as Bor (1991) points out, they are at the forefront of professional caregiving to patients and families affected with or by AIDS. If AIDS continues to increase in incidence (and there is every evidence that it will), then health care professionals will find themselves caring for more and more people who have developed a range of infections. At least two things follow from this. All health care professionals must have a considerable knowledge about the nature of AIDS. They will also have to explore their own values and attitudes to the problem and develop counselling strategies and skills.

On the first issue, the question of health care professionals developing their knowledge base, the problem is a difficult one. Just as the AIDS virus itself seems to be changing (Connor and Kingman, 1990), so does the research and knowledge base. No worker in the field can expect to stay completely up to date. On the other hand, certain issues stay the same. The mode of transmission of the virus is well documented and everyone should have a clear idea about what constitutes safe sex and what to do to avoid contracting AIDS (Miller, 1987, 1990).

In summary of the issues involved in HIV/AIDS counselling, Sketchley (1989) suggests that counselling people with AIDS involves three domains:

- educational issues;
- advice;
- psychosocial issues.

The worried well

This is not a particularly comfortable expression but it has been used to describe people who do not suffer from a particular disease or disorder but who are, nevertheless, worried about themselves. Green and Davey (1992) suggest that, in the early days of AIDS counselling, many who sought advice fell into this category.

The worried well are not a homogeneous group. They can range from people who are edging towards what some psychiatrists might call 'neurosis' to people who simply want to know what they should do about aspects of their lives. Traditionally, the worried well have been given little sympathy from medical and health care professionals, who would prefer to deal with frank illness or tangible problems. It is important, however, not to 'pathologize' further the person who is both worried and well. The label should not become a diagnosis.

Perhaps the main point is that the worried well should be taken seriously. They are as entitled as anyone else to be listened to and given appropriate help. Trivialization or glib reassurance that 'everything will work out OK' or that 'there is nothing to worry about' falls well short of the sort of help that people are seeking. Once again, the key word seems to be *listening*. If we can listen to the worried and well person, we may help to alleviate some of the worry and to ensure that they remain well. Sickness or disability is not a prerequisite for seeking counselling.

AIDS counselling in adolescence and childhood

The prevention of the spread of HIV/AIDS may depend, in the West, on the appropriate education and counselling of children and adolescents. Hein (1989) has suggested that there are important differences between adolescents and adults in sexual behaviour and AIDS epidemiology that should be considered in planning appropriate responses to the AIDS epidemic. The differences are as follows.

- A higher percentage of adolescent cases is acquired by heterosexual transmission;
- a higher percentage of infected adolescents is asymptomatic;
- a higher percentage of infected adolescents are minorities;
- special ethical and legal considerations pertain to minors;
- adolescents differ from adults in sociocognitive reasoning;
- there are special economic and medical implications for infected adolescents who are pregnant;
- unified community support systems for infected adolescents are not available;
- adolescents as a population include a higher percentage of 'sexual adventurers', who have many sexual contacts and rarely use contraceptives;
- convenient and appropriate health services are relatively unavailable for adolescents.

Health professionals who counsel young people in this field are likely to find some differences between what adolescents *know* about HIV/AIDS and what they *do*.

> ***Surveys of sexual activity among high school students and among college students conducted since the AIDS epidemic indicate that a higher percentage of youths engage in unsafe sexual activity in spite of having a high level of knowledge about AIDS and about the value of condoms in protecting against HIV infections. (Henggeler et al., 1992).***

Added to all this is the controversy that has surrounded the teaching of young people identified as HIV positive. Often, it would seem, the counsellor of young people in this field needs to consider the attitudes of parents, teachers and other people who come into contact with children and adolescents. Gostin (1990) summarizes some of the emotive attitudes that have been observed in this area.

> ***From the earliest times of the HIV epidemic, exclusion of school children infected with HIV from their classrooms was an issue debated with great emotion. Parents of children infected with HIV sued school boards for denying children state education, giving homebound instruction, or making the child wait for inordinate periods while the board developed a policy. In other cases, HIV-infected children were permitted to attend school, but they were clearly singled out as different by being placed alone in a separate 'modular' classroom, by being required to use a separate bathroom and to be accompanied by an adult on all field trips, or even being isolated inside a glass booth.***

Clearly, the whole area of counselling children and adolescents about HIV/AIDS is a complicated one. The health professional as counsellor needs to know not only about the syndrome, modes of infection and means of prevention but about children, adolescents and their ways of viewing and operating in the world. Counselling in this area calls for all the skills described so far in this book and, further, for particular and accurate knowledge.

AIDS counselling for health care professionals

Many courses in AIDS counselling are already available to both health care professionals and other carers. The question remains, however, whether all health care professionals should undergo some basic training in the field. At the moment, it is for individual health care professionals to identify their own needs and wants. It is questionable how long this state of affairs can be allowed to continue. If, as is suspected, the incidence of AIDS continues to grow, the AIDS issue is going to be everyone's business. In the meantime, more research needs to be undertaken to establish how best to train health care professionals in helping those with AIDS.

From a review of the literature, three elements of training appear to be important:

- information about AIDS;
- values clarification;
- counselling skills.

Any training programme for health care professionals would need to include these elements. First, health care professionals need up-to-date and accurate information about the prevention, incidence, nature and characteristics of AIDS and HIV. They also need information about the psychosocial issues involved in being a person with AIDS.

Values clarification is an approach to helping people to explore their beliefs, values and attitudes (Kirschenbaum, 1978). Again, these should be examined before health care professionals start working in the capacity of AIDS counsellors.

Finally, given that the focus of the role is counselling, a grounding in basic counselling skills is essential to any programme of this sort. The skills of questioning, reflecting, empathy building and checking for understanding can be augmented by skills in confrontation and effective information giving (Heron, 1986; Nelson-Jones, 1995). Whilst, as we have noted, the approach in AIDS counselling may not always be client centred, client centred skills can serve as the basis of a broader range of effective counselling skills.

Emotions and AIDS

Given that individuals vary in their response to life-threatening situations, it is difficult to generalize about the ways in which people react to the knowledge that they are HIV positive or have AIDS. George (1989), however, identifies the following emotions that he suggests are frequently associated with the experience of having AIDS.

- Shock;
- relief;
- anger;
- guilt;
- decreased self-esteem;
- loss of identity;
- loss of a sense of security;
- loss of personal control;
- fear of what may happen in the future;
- sadness and depressed mood;
- obsessions and compulsions;
- positive adjustment.

This list could be easily added to. It is notable that only one of George's items is positive and he suggests that positive adjustment to the realization of having AIDS may occur with little intervention from professionals. This suggests that the AIDS counsellor may well have to face a wide range of negative emotions.

COUNSELLING CHILDREN

'Counselling', in this context, may be too strong a term. I prefer to use the expression 'talking with children'. Many people, for a variety of reasons, find that quite difficult. For some, children seem to be 'different' from adults: they are smaller, they talk a different language and it seems a long time since the adult listener was their age. However, children need to be able to talk and need, very much, someone they can trust and have listen to them.

Principles from the world of counselling may shed light on how we might begin to think about helping children*. 'Adult' counselling usually involves two people: the counsellor and the client. The counsellor is usually the person who asks questions, reflects back feelings and thoughts and checks that they have understood what the client has said. In the client centred tradition of counselling, it is taken as given that it is the client who will find their own solutions to their problems. There seems no immediate reason why such an approach cannot be used in communicating with children. The main point of helping children should be to allow those children to express their thoughts and feelings and to identify strategies for dealing with difficulties – whatever those 'difficulties' might be.

There are numerous occasions on which children may need to talk through difficulties and problems. Examples include: prior to surgical or

* I am indebted to my friend and colleague, Jim Richardson, for his help and advice on talking to children.

medical intervention; in coming to terms with acute or chronic illness or disability; following the death of a parent, relative or close friend or after another family crisis has occurred; or in coming to terms with new, anxiety-provoking ideas and realizations revealed to the child during his developmental progress. Whether or not all these situations would be deemed 'counselling' situations is not the point: the basic skills of counselling apply to them all. The person who listens and helps children is already functioning in the role of a counsellor.

The literature often identifies *listening* as the most important skill in communicating effectively with other people (Calnan, 1983; Egan, 1990; Tschudin, 1991). The ability to sit and listen to a child as they talk through what is happening to them is the starting point of any therapeutic relationship. In many situations, the mere fact of being heard is all that is required. In other situations, help and advice will be appropriate. Whilst the client centred approach has been widely advocated as appropriate to helping adults, it is possible that if information giving is necessary as part of this process for children, they may need more direction and prescription. In the end, though, like adults, children have to come to terms with their problems in their own individual ways. Like adults, no-one can make a decision about a problem *for* a child: they have to make their own decisions in their own time. However, there are certain issues that can help in the process of offering counselling to children. An understanding of the processes and peculiarities of the development in childhood can help in the evolution of empathy and in the skill of listening.

Issues in communicating with children

Children's communication abilities vary with their age and experience (Prosser, 1985). The health care professional must be sensitive not only to subtle non-verbal communication but also to sometimes idiosyncratic use of language. In particular, children may have unusual ways of describing situations or feelings for which they do not yet have the language. An example of this is the child who was asked to describe her pain and referred to it as 'like a sausage' (Jerrett and Evans, 1986). It is important to try to get 'inside' the child's frame of reference and to try to understand what *they* mean by the words they use. This calls for considerable empathy: a quality that Rogers (1957) identified as a necessary and sufficient condition for therapeutic change. Empathizing with children may be more difficult than with adults: it is certainly just as essential. Children's interpersonal responses are influenced by their interpretation of the context and situation. This may, in the light of adult logic, be quite unexpectedly different from an adult's interpretation.

Children's dependence on their parents/carers may mean that, particularly when they feel frightened or vulnerable, they might prefer to communicate with a stranger obliquely, e.g. via a parent. A fine distinction is drawn between treating the child as an individual on the one hand and as an enmeshed member of a supportive family on the other (Jackson and Vessey, 1992). None of us exists in isolation. We are all closely bound up with the lives of the people with whom we live and work. For the child, the ego boundary – the difference between 'me here' and 'you out there' – may be even less pronounced than is the case with adults.

Children have a tendency towards literal, concrete communication. Witticisms, sarcasms and word games may be lost on the child, clouding communication. Again, Carl Rogers saw the ability to be concrete in dealing with others as an essential feature of the counselling process.

Most family members use a 'shorthand' when talking to each other. Family names, for example, may not be 'proper' names. Often, too, families develop secret or private languages (Crystal, 1987) through which to communicate. There may, for example, be family words for certain meals, for drinks or for certain events. The genesis of these names may be lost in family history. More importantly, the child may not know that this is a family word and may think that everyone uses language in this way. It is important for the person who talks to a child to clarify any unusual use of language in order to have a more complete understanding of any given situation.

Indirect communication, perhaps using a doll or a soft toy, may be successful with the shy or wary child as this diffuses the focus from the child and introduces an element of play and therefore normality. A child at a stage of development characterized by animistic or magical thinking will find this form of communication natural.

Paralinguistic devices such as variations in the speed, rhythm, tone and volume of speech as well as extra 'padding' words such as 'um', 'ah' and 'well', which have little direct meaning, are extensively used by adults and may be misinterpreted by children. When children do begin to use these communication styles they may do so inexpertly and this in turn may be awkward for adults to understand.

To make communication between adults and children as effective as possible, it is important that the adult firmly establishes what the child's understanding is of the issue in question. This is particularly important when the discussion centres on an abstraction about which the child may have no experience. An example of this is the topic of death; if the child has an inaccurate perception of what death is, he may find it extremely difficult to understand an adult-level conversation on this topic (Lansdown, 1992). Effective talking with the child can only occur when the adult is clear about the terms which are understandable to the child on the basis of his experience and stage of cognitive development.

Avoid rushing the child – allow him a little time to get to know you. Let him dictate the pace. The flustered child is unlikely to be able to – or want to – talk with the adult who is pressurizing him. Watch the child for signs of tiredness and withdrawal; in these circumstances communication is less likely to succeed.

It was acknowledged in Chapter 1 that many adults want some form of spiritual counselling and that this may or may not take on a religious connotation. What is less commonly recognized is children's need for talking about spiritual matters.

Practical guidelines for talking to children

From the above issues and from the considerable literature on counselling and talking with children, the following guidelines may be identified.

- Listen to the child; although his message may not be immediately clear, he has much to say (Coles, 1992).
- Find out what the child likes to be called. Do not assume that he will like you to call him by a nickname or a name used in the family. Give the child your own name – introduce yourself!
- Be aware of levels and stages of child development. This can help you to pitch your questions and responses at the correct level. Observe the child's response for signs of success in this.
- Respond to the child as an individual. Do not assume that 'all children are much the same'. Children are complete human beings in their own right. When meeting a child for the first time, the only thing that you can assume is that you are about to meet a new person.
- Talk to children 'normally': do not talk down to them or patronize them and be aware of over use of endearments such as 'dear' or 'love'. Try to keep speech clear, avoid very erudite words and expressions. Keep sentences short. Repeat/rephrase as necessary/ based on response.
- Respect the child. Remember that he is a human being just like you, only a little younger.
- Think about the environment in which you talk to the child. If you are working in a hospital or clinical setting, find a quiet room in which to talk; children's wards and outpatients departments are often excruciatingly noisy places. Alternatively, talk as you play with the child.
- Use play to communicate with smaller children.
- Do not try to copy children's slang or adopt their mannerisms. I recall a conversation with my adolescent son in which I tried to use some of the slang that he used with his friends. His suggestion was: 'You shouldn't even try, because even when you get the words right, it doesn't sound right.' 'Why?' 'Because you're too old.'
- Believe children. Trust must be the basis of any relationship and it is particularly important with children.
- Remember that most children are taught not to talk to strangers. Therefore, some children will prefer talking to you only in the company of one of their parents. Do not assume that children will want to talk to you. Also, as Shapiro (1984) suggests:

> ***Children are used to being talked about by people who care for them; it happens all the time with their parents, and they can accept this as a part of life. They do not necessarily distrust the therapist who also talks to their parents, as long as the therapist's intentions are made clear from the beginning of the treatment.***

- Allow the child to determine the issue of proximity. Do not stand or sit too close to them or automatically put your arm around them. Allow the child to decide on these issues. Be aware of what might, for the child, constitute a threat. Sometimes, it is necessary to be creative and to find out where the child would like to sit and talk. In her excellent book *Children and Counselling*, Margaret Crompton (1992) writes as follows about the issue of where to counsel children.

> ***. . . Yet somewhere can always be found. During my work with children in 1989–90, I carried materials in a large shopping bag. Since it was not possible to work with Mark in his foster home and there was no office within miles, I met him once a week from school and asked: 'Where shall we go today?' The answer was always the same, despite the possibility of an interesting castle and an inviting river: 'To the café.'***

Crompton's book is essential reading for anyone either considering a career working with children or who needs further information about counselling and talking with children.

Talking to children is an activity which many adults will undertake without hesitation. With a little attention to some ground rules, the likelihood of successful communication can be maximized and the potential for this activity to offer benefit, comfort and pleasure to both the child and the adult can be safeguarded. The key to success lies in the adult's appreciation of the various facets of the child as a dynamic, developing human being with sometimes imperfect, unpractised psychological, social and communication skills. Everyday communication with children merges subtly with counselling – communication with a therapeutic purpose (Macleod Clark *et al.*, 1991). With practice in the basic skills of talking to children, you should come to recognize when basic skills are no longer sufficient and specialist counselling assistance is required. This will signal the need for referral. Thus, familiarity with the ground rules of communicating with children may help you to recognize your own limitations in this field.

Street (1989), in discussing the question of family counselling, suggests that the following four questions need to be asked of families that present for counselling. The questions impinge directly on the process of talking to children in therapeutic settings.

- Does the family have information on which to base an appropriate view of the task?
- Is the communication in the family clear and open or does it need to be clarified?
- Is it possible to specify the needs of everyone in the family?
- What negotiations for adaptions to change need to be made?

OTHER CONTEXTS

This chapter has only hinted at the variety of arenas in which counselling may take place. Many others exist. There has been debate, for instance, about race. Lago and Thompson (1989) suggest that the following may be the major themes in this field.

- In order to understand the relationships between black and white people today, a knowledge of the history of differing racial groups is required.
- Counsellors also require an understanding of how current society works in relation to race, the exercise of power, the effects of discrimination, stereotyping, how ideologies sabotage policies and so on.
- Counsellors require a personal awareness of where they stand in relation to these issues.

Other writers have discussed the issues of sexual orientation (Beane, 1981; Lourea, 1985) and sexual dysfunction (Bancroft, 1983; Fairburn *et al.*, 1983). Yet others have described the particular issues involved in counselling the unemployed and those who need career guidance (Ball, 1984; Hopson, 1985). The literature on sexuality counselling is considerable and those who need further information about job-related counselling are referred to the various journals on the topic, which include the *British Journal of Guidance and Counselling* and *Employee Counselling Today*. Other contexts which may involve the giving of clear information are identified in Dryden *et al.* (1989) and include the following.

- Pastoral counselling;
- counselling in death and bereavement;
- counselling people with disabilities and chronic illnesses;
- counselling people with alcohol and drug problems.

The range of counselling situations remains vast. Indeed, it may be argued that the term 'counselling' is also an umbrella term for a wide range of varied activities carried out by a number of different sorts of professionals. Within that spectrum, the full range of counselling approaches from the client centred to the confronting may be found.

10 Problems and support in counselling

Counselling takes time and energy on the part of the counsellor. The fact of being intimately involved in someone else's world means that both counsellor and client form a close and sometimes painful relationship. If counselling is to be successful, it will involve change on the part of the client. It may also involve change on the part of the counsellor. Most of us resist change – we prefer to stay as we are. In counselling, it often seems as though the client wants problem resolution without having to change himself! Clearly, life problems cannot change without the person who experiences them changing too. The nature of the counselling relationship, then, is one that develops, regresses, modulates and is finally outgrown. Along that dimension, various difficulties can arise and in this chapter a number of such problems are identified and explored.

Confidentiality

Should what is said in a counselling situation remain confidential? On the face of it, the answer seems fairly straightforward: that in usual circumstances, what the client tells the counsellor should remain only with those two people. On the other hand, the client may disclose things that the counsellor feels must be passed on another person. Examples of such situations might include the following.

- The person who says that she is going to kill herself.
- The client who tells the counsellor that he is abusing one of his children.
- The person who seems, in the counsellor's opinion, to be showing signs of mental illness.

Such situations call for considerable soul searching on the part of the counsellor. Various possible equations can be worked out for anticipating and coping with the question of confidentiality in counselling.

- The counsellor may offer total confidentiality to the client. In this case, the counsellor must be prepared to stick to their word and *everything* that is said must remain confidential. One of the considerable strengths of the Samaritan movement is that it offers this level of confidentiality. On the other hand, the health professional is often in a different situation from a Samaritan and is accountable to the health care organization in which they work. It may be debatable whether or not such total confidentiality can be offered by a health care professional.

- The counsellor may tell the client at the beginning of the relationship that the relationship will not be a confidential one and that certain people may have to know about the content of counselling conversations. This is the reverse side of the previous option. Whilst some clients may feel that this lack of confidentiality is inhibiting, at least the contract between the two people is clear. Also, the client can be reassured that people will only be given information on a 'need to know' basis.
- The counsellor may avoid discussing the question of confidentiality as an issue in its own right but consult the client, during the relationship, as to the degree to which that person is comfortable about information being shared with other professional colleagues.

Sometimes, of course, the nature of the content of a counselling relationship is not of the 'confidential' sort. Some conversations do not contain very much 'personal' information but many do. All health professionals working as counsellors need to address and face the issue of confidentiality in counselling. Munro *et al.* (1989) offer these other useful guidelines.

- The client should know where she stands in relation to confidentiality. For example, if case discussion is routine within an agency, the client should be told this.
- Where referral to another agency or consultation with another family member seems appropriate, the client's prior permission should be sought.
- When a client specifically requests confidentiality regarding a particular disclosure, this must be respected.
- Where confidentiality has to be broken because of the law or because of danger to the client's life, she should be informed as soon as possible.
- Records of interviews should be minimal, noting only what is essential within the particular agency setting. Records should be locked up, shared only with authorized recipients who would also be bound by confidentiality, and destroyed when the counselling relationship is terminated.
- An atmosphere of confidentiality is even more important than any verbal reassurance of it. If, for example, during the interview note taking is considered essential, the counsellor could offer to let the client see what is being written or even write it herself.
- Confidentiality, when part of a professional code of ethics, should be upheld.

Carrying someone else's confidential thoughts and feelings can be painful and distracting. When someone shares an important, personal and even dangerous thought or feeling, part of the responsibility that goes with it is transferred to the person who receives it. If, for example, I tell you that I am planning to kill myself, the fact that you now know this means that you have to decide whether or not you (as another human being) are responsible for doing something about it. Also, you have to consider whether or not you *can* do anything about it. A person who sets themselves up as a counsellor must be prepared to shoulder other people's problems. It is not simply a question of sitting and listening, noting what the other person says and moving on. When we hear intimate thoughts and feelings, they stay with us. If the relationship is not a confidential one, we can sometimes share that burden with other colleagues. If we remain in a totally confidential relationship, then we must be prepared to live with whatever we hear.

TRANSFERENCE AND COUNTERTRANSFERENCE

As the client discloses himself to the counsellor, so an element of dependence creeps into the relationship. Because the counsellor is accepting of what the client has to say, the client may begin to cast the counsellor in the role of a person from the past who has also adopted this accepting, allowing position: a trusted parent. Transference refers to the client's coming to view the counsellor as if they were the all-forgiving, positive parent. As a result, the client may come to view the counsellor as one of the most important people in his life.

Countertransference, on the other hand, refers to the feelings that the counsellor develops for the client. Usually, these are positive in nature and fed by the positive feelings that the client expresses for the counsellor. A problem arises, however, if the counsellor does not notice that she is being cast in the 'good parent' role and begins unawares to play 'mother' (or 'father') to the client's 'son' (or 'daughter'). What happens then is that old child/parent relationships are played out and little progress is achieved. The counsellor unconsciously colludes with the role that the client has cast her in and the relationship staggers on until either the client finds little reward in it and discovers that the counsellor is 'only human' after all or the counsellor finds the whole thing too claustrophobic and releases herself from it.

Two practical approaches may be taken to the question of transference and countertransference. One is that the counsellor learns to notice what happens as the relationship develops and looks out for growing dependence on the part of the client. As the dependence develops, the counsellor can encourage the client to also become aware of it and make the counselling relationship itself the subject of discussion. Thus a joint focus is maintained in the counselling sessions: the client's life problems and the counsellor/client relationship. Much can be learned from the latter that will help with the former, for the quality of the client/counsellor relationship can reflect other relationships the client may have. It is as though the client/ counsellor relationship represents one, intense example of how the client relates to other people in everyday life.

The second approach to dealing with transference and countertransference is for the counsellor to have an experienced colleague acting as supervisor, with whom the counselling relationship can be discussed confidentially and who may offer suggestions as to how she sees the counselling developing. Thus another, arguably objective, point of view is offered which may enable the counsellor to gain a little more objectivity. Three types of 'contract' may be used in the counsellor/supervisor relationship.

1 The supervisor agrees only to listen to the counsellor, talking through her difficulties in the counselling relationship.
2 The supervisor agrees to make occasional comments as the counsellor talks.
3 The supervisor agrees to make intensive interventions during the conversation and may act in a 'devil's advocate' capacity to explore, in detail, the relationship that the counsellor has built up with the client.

These three contracts, agreed at the beginning of the counsellor/client relationship, can determine the degree of involvement that the supervisor has. Obviously, at any time, the contract can be changed to meet the altering needs of the counsellor.

At regular meetings with a supervisor, the counsellor can work through the sometimes painful period of the counsellor/client relationship in which transference is at its most acute.

Another basis for counsellor/supervisor meetings is for the counsellor to write out the counsellor/client dialogue, after the counselling session, as she remembers it. This then serves as a basis for counsellor/supervisor discussions and can also help in identifying the counsellor's growing skill in using counselling interventions effectively.

The supervisor's role in the relationship is not as 'counselling expert' but as one who listens and perhaps offers her perception of what is going on between counsellor and client. No counsellor gets to the point where they do not 'need' a supervisor. The support offered by such a person is useful to the health practitioner who is just beginning a counselling role and also to the expert who has had many years experience.

Transference in practice

Geoff is an occupational therapist in a unit aiming to rehabilitate those with long-term psychiatric illnesses, in a large psychiatric hospital. He is trying to encourage the development of effective social skills with a small group of five patients and organizes role modelling, practice and reinforcement of socially acceptable behaviour. He finds one, younger, patient very difficult to cope with and begins to feel that he does not like that patient. He allows the situation to continue for some time but finds himself becoming increasingly hostile towards the young man. Finally, Geoff is able to talk through his feelings with the Head OT, with whom he has a good relationship. The Head OT, who has had counselling training, is able to explore with Geoff what it is that makes the young patient so unacceptable to Geoff. During the course of their conversations, it becomes apparent that the young man reminds Geoff partly of himself as a younger person and partly of his younger brother, with whom he had never got on. The identification of this 'transference' relationship allows Geoff to explore ways in which the young patient is different from both Geoff and his brother. In this way, Geoff becomes able to 'disidentify' with the associations he had made and to see the patient more clearly for his own strengths and weaknesses. Geoff is able to return to the social skills group and work with the young man in more constructive ways.

DEALING WITH 'BLOCKS' IN COUNSELLING

Periodically, in many counselling relationships, a point may be reached where the client appears to be making little progress and the relationship seems to be 'stuck'. At least two practical approaches may be taken to this problem. First, the counsellor can acknowledge to the client that she perceives the relationship to be 'stuck' and thus verbalizes and makes explicit what has previously only been hinted at. This in itself can serve to push the relationship on and open up discussion on other things that are not being talked about. Sometimes the block is caused, unknowingly, by the counsellor herself. If the client is discussing a problem that is also a problem for the counsellor, then the counsellor may skirt round the issue rather than face it. Few of us like our own unresolved problems brought out into the open, particularly by someone else! This highlights further the need for the prospective counsellor to develop self-awareness and to explore some of her own life problems before helping others to tackle theirs.

A second approach to dealing with blocks is to allow or even encourage the block to remain unresolved. This paradoxical way of working can sometimes be particularly effective. It is as though, if we allow the problem to exist, then problem resolution is encouraged. On the other hand, the more we fight blocks, the more they continue to be a problem. Facing up to, accepting and 'staying with' the block can be a productive means of allowing the relationship to develop. Sometimes, the longer we can stay confused about where the relationship is going, the more successful the outcome.

COPING WITH SILENCE

There are many occasions on which the counselling relationship falls into silence. There are different sorts of silences, from the meditative, thoughtful silence through to the hostile, angry silence. It is important that the counsellor learns to differentiate between the sort of silence in which a counsellor intervention is called for and the sort of silence in which the client is quietly thinking things through. Normally, when the client is 'asking' for the counsellor to say something, he will make eye contact with her and look towards her. When he is thinking about things his eyes will usually be defocused or, sometimes, looking upwards (Bandler and Grinder, 1982). It is important that the counsellor does not 'overtalk' because of anxiety about the silence. It is tempting to imagine that every silence needs filling and if the client isn't talking, then the counsellor should! Thoughtful silences are often the most productive aspects of counselling. However, occasionally it is helpful for the counsellor to ask: 'What are you thinking?' or 'What's the thought?'. These are particularly useful when the client suddenly falls silent or stops his train of conversation and glances to one side. Often these are indicators of sudden insight which may be usefully verbalized.

CONFRONTATION IN COUNSELLING

There are times when the counselling relationship cannot be purely client centred. Sometimes the counsellor needs to draw attention to particular behaviours or beliefs that are negatively affecting the client's life. There are times, too, when we have to confront the client with bad news: news of a sudden death, for example. At other times, we need to be able to tell the client of the effect they are having on us.

The prospect of confrontation often causes anxiety. Two classic ways in which a counsellor may react to that anxiety are outlined by Heron (1986) (Figure 10.1). He describes two extremes: the 'pussyfooting' approach, where the counsellor skirts gently all round the topic but never comes to the point, and the 'sledgehammer' approach, where the counsellor allows her anxiety about confrontation to build up to the point where it is all blurted out in one go and may degenerate to the point where a verbal attack is made on the client. This, perhaps, is a version of the 'last straw syndrome', described in Chapter 8. Neither approach is very effective. A more constructive approach is the assertive, confronting approach in which the counsellor clearly and quietly states what it is they want to confront the client on and remains ready, if necessary, to repeat the confrontation. Such repetition may be necessary because there can be no guarantee how the client will react to clear, assertive confrontation. Some people respond by becoming submissive and quiet. The temptation, here, may be to 'back off' and to withdraw the confrontation. On the other hand, some people respond by becoming angry and again (though for different reasons) the counsellor may feel tempted to withdraw. The most effective approach, however, is to stay with the confrontation and to ensure that it is heard. A note of caution needs to be sounded, however, in that it is easy for the counsellor to 'overtalk' in these situations and to overstate the confrontation because of the anxiety generated by the task. Effective confrontation usually involves the confrontation being made and then time allowed for it to sink in.

Another approach to confrontation is the 'sandwich' approach. Three stages are involved in this method. In the first stage (or the 'top slice of the sandwich'), warning of the confrontation is given by the counsellor to the client. This is immediately followed up by the confrontation itself (the 'filling of the sandwich'). The third stage involves the counsellor offering the client support, without withdrawing the confrontation in any way (the

Figure 10:1

Confrontation and its variants.

Aggressive	Confronting	Submissive
'Sledgehammer' approach: the counsellor becomes aggressive and interventions become an attack on the person.	'Confronting' approach: the counsellor stays calm, keeps to the point and is prepared to repeat his or her confronting statement.	'Pussyfooting' approach: the counsellor is vague, unclear and has a tendency to go 'round the houses'.

'bottom layer of the sandwich'). An example of this in action is as follows, where the counsellor has to give the client news of a relative's death.

Counsellor: I have some very bad news for you. I'm sorry to tell you that your mother died earlier this afternoon. I know it will be a great shock to you and I want you to know that I will stay with you.

What are the principles behind the sandwich approach? First, the 'warning' that comes before the confrontation allows the client to anticipate the coming confrontation. It is important, however, that the confronting statement follows almost immediately, so that the client does not have to imagine, for too long, what form the confrontation will take. The final layer of the sandwich offers the client some means of support after experiencing the confrontation. Notice that in this offering of very bad news, the language used is completely unambiguous. It is vital, when breaking bad news, that there can be no doubt as to the meaning of the confrontation. Thus, all euphemisms should be avoided for the sake of clarity.

The sandwich approach in action

Joe is a social worker with a caseload that covers a large housing estate. He is asked by his Director to follow up a report that has been sent in by a local school teacher that suggests that one of the children in her class may have received non-accidental injuries in the home. Joe visits the child's house and meets his parents. His first task is to develop rapport with the parents and he does this by introducing himself and by discussing his role and by then discreetly asking the parents about themselves. He follows this, directly, by suggesting that he has some difficult issues to talk about and moves straight into outlining what those issues are. He then offers the parents the chance to talk things through in detail, to establish their reactions to the accusations. He then 'backs off' and allows the parents to react to the report, having used the 'sandwich' method of breaking difficult and upsetting news to the parents.

This approach can be used in a variety of confronting contexts. Examples of the sorts of situations in which the counsellor may be required to confront the client include the following.

- When the counsellor has to give the client difficult or shocking information (e.g. death of a relative, notice of a diagnosis, challenging in suspected cases of child abuse).
- When the client is using compulsive, negative self-statements (e.g. 'I'll never be able to walk again . . .' 'I've never been any good at anything . . .'
- When the client is using 'games' in the relationship and manipulating the counsellor (e.g the 'Yes, but' game, where the client answers every suggestion the counsellor makes with the phrase 'Yes, I would, but . . .'. For further details of this sort of game playing, see Berne (1964), Harris (1969) and James and Jongeward (1971).
- When contractual issues need to be clarified (e.g. previously agreed times of meeting and of finishing the counselling sessions).
- When 'excuses' need to be challenged. Wheeler and Janis (1980) identify the following sorts of excuses that a client may use:
  - *complacency*: the 'it won't happen to me' attitude;
  - *rationalization*: the 'it's not as bad as it looks' approach;
  - *procrastination*: the 'nothing needs to be done at the moment' argument;
  - *passing the buck*: The 'I'm not the one who needs to do something' idea.

Arguably, all of these excuses may have to be confronted at various stages in certain counselling relationships. Care needs to be taken, however, that counselling of this sort does not degenerate into heavy-handed patronage of the client by the counsellor.

Of all the aspects of counselling, perhaps effective confrontation is the most difficult and needs the most practice. It is worth reflecting on how you handle confrontation!

Confrontation in practice

Julia is a speech therapist working with a young child, Clare, who has hearing problems. During one of their appointments, Clare's mother begins to tell Julia of Clare's difficult behaviour at home and is very critical of the child. She does this with the child sitting in front of both Julia and her mother. Julia reaches out and gently holds the mother's arm and says 'I would appreciate it if we could talk about this in a few minutes when Clare goes in to see the doctor'. The mother, however, continues to talk negatively about her daughter. Julia repeats: 'I want to stop you and suggest that we talk in a few minutes'. After a third repetition of the request by Julia, Clare's mother stops talking but is encouraged to talk more freely when her daughter is not present. At a later appointment, Julia, Clare and her mother are more easily able to talk freely between themselves. Clare's mother has been able to 'offload' to Julia, without hurting her daughter's feelings.

In the instance described here, Julia has confronted the mother and used the 'broken record' method to ensure that what she wanted to say got through. 'Broken record' refers to the technique of calmly repeating the confronting statement until it is 'heard'.

THE LIMITS OF COUNSELLING

Much of the counselling that health professionals will be involved in will concern what may be called the 'worried well': people who have particular life problems but who are essentially mentally well. Whilst the question of where 'wellness' ends and mental illness begins is by no means clearcut, the health professional should always bear in mind her limitations. It is tempting, once we have established a close relationship with another person, to believe that we alone can help them. Sometimes it is with extreme reluctance that we call in other advice or help. It is, however, important that we only take on relationships that we can handle and in which we can be therapeutic. The health professional working as counsellor may not be able to adequately help the following types of clients.

- The person who is clinically depressed and talking of suicide.
- The person who is hallucinating or deluded.
- The person who has an organic mental illness.
- The person whose behaviour is potentially dangerous to themselves or others.

Making judgements about when to counsel and when to refer to another agency is always difficult and it is helpful if the practitioner can talk through, in confidence, the problems of the person whom she feels may benefit from further referral. Referrals for psychiatric help are normally made through the person's general practitioner or sometimes through occupational health agencies.

Perhaps more difficult is persuading the client that you are not the best person to help them. Suggesting referral to other agencies may be seen either as a rebuff or as a sign that you view them as being seriously mentally ill. Bearing in mind the discussion above regarding confrontation, the person who cannot be helped through counselling must be approached about the possibility of referral: to do otherwise is to limit the possibilities that person has of regaining his health.

BURNOUT

The process of counselling and of coping with others can take its toll on the counsellor and health professional. The word 'burnout' (derived from the idea that once a rocket has burnt up its fuel it is then of no use but it continues to circulate in space) has been used to denote the overall feeling that a person can experience when exhausted by being intimately involved in human relationships. Gerard Corey (cited by Murgatroyd, 1986) lists a number of causes of burnout which the counsellor and health professional needs to bear in mind if she is to avoid it.

- Doing the same type of helping over and over again with little variation.
- Giving a great deal of one's own emotional and personal energy to others whilst getting very little back.
- Being under a constant pressure to produce results in a certain time scale when the time scale and the pressure are unrealistic.
- Working with a difficult group: for example, those who are highly resistant to change, those who have been 'sent' for help but who do not wish to be helped or those for whom the chances of change are small because of the nature of their difficulties (for example, the terminally ill).
- The absence of support from immediate colleagues and an abundance of criticism – what might be called 'the atmosphere of certain doubt'.
- Lack of trust between those who engage in helping and those who manage the organizational resources that make helping possible – a feature sometimes present in voluntary organizations.
- Not having the opportunity to take new directions, to develop one's own approach or to experiment with new models of working – being unnecessarily constrained.
- Having few opportunities for training, continuing education, supervision or support.
- Unresolved personal conflicts beyond the helping and counselling work which interfere with the helper's ability to be effective, for example, marital problems, health problems.

Burnout in practice

Ann is a district nurse working mainly with elderly patients. Recently, her caseload has increased and she has also taken on an Open University course. Her eldest child, who is 11, is having difficulty settling at his new secondary school. Ann slowly finds that she is losing interest in the elderly people that she is visiting. She also finds that she is avoiding working on her Open University assignments and she begins to wonder how she had ever been interested in the course at all. Her general disenchantment is brought to a head when she visits a younger patient who begins to tell her about her marital problems. Ann realizes that she has no interest at all in what the woman has to say and just wants to leave the house.

Later, Ann discontinues her Open University course and begins to consider whether or not she should remain a district nurse. She is suffering from 'burnout'. It is only after she has had a number of long talks with her husband that she realizes the degree of emotional exhaustion that she has been experiencing. It is only then that her husband also begins to realize how difficult life has become for her. Together, they map out a plan to reorganize family life a little, so that Ann has some 'time for herself'. Her husband agrees to take over more of the household chores and both Ann and her husband find time to sit down and listen to their son talk about his problems at school. She does not go back to the Open University course but enrols instead at a local evening class. Slowly, her interest in her work returns and she feels less afraid to talk about the negative feelings she sometimes has.

It is unreasonable to suppose that we can continue to work with and for others without paying attention to our own needs. The person who wants to avoid burnout needs to consider at least the following preventive measures.

- Vary your work as much as possible.
- Consider your education and training needs and plan ahead.
- Take care of your physical health.
- Consider new ways of developing counselling skills and try them out.
- Develop an effective supervision or peer support system.
- Nurture your friendships and relationships with others.
- Develop a range of interests away from work.
- Attend 'refresher' workshops occasionally, as a means of 'updating' and also as a means of experiencing new ideas and methods.
- Initiate your own projects, without relying on others to approve them.
- Seek positive and reliable feedback on your performance from other people.

PEER SUPPORT: CO-COUNSELLING

If we are to avoid burnout and subsequent disillusionment with the task of counselling, it is vital that we have an adequate peer support system. Co-counselling offers one such means of ensuring that two people regularly review their life situation and their counselling practice.

Co-counselling was originally devised by Harvey Jackins in the USA (Jackins, 1965, 1970) and further developed by John Heron in the UK (Heron, 1978). Basically, it involves two people who have trained as co-counsellors meeting on a regular basis for two hours. For the first hour, one of the partners is 'counsellor' or helper and the other is 'client' or talker. In the second hour, roles are reversed and the 'counsellor' becomes the 'client' and vice versa. The 'counselling' role in co-counselling, however, is not the traditional role of counsellor: the role demands more that the person listens and gives attention to their partner than would usually be the case. In this respect, co-counselling offers a bonus to the practising counsellor in that it is an excellent way of developing and enhancing listening skills. In its most basic form, the hour spent in the role of 'counsellor' is one of listening only, while the client verbally reviews any aspect of their life that they choose: their emotional status, life problems, recent difficulties, future plans and so forth. An important aspect of co-counselling is that what is talked about during the co-counselling sessions is not discussed away from the session. For this reason, it is helpful if the two people meet only for co-counselling. To this end, co-counselling 'networks' have been set up which enable those trained to contact others.

Having the sustained and supportive attention of another person can be very liberating. It can create the circumstances in which a person is truly able to work things out for herself. Whilst the co-counselling format allows for certain verbal interventions on the part of the 'counsellor', these never extend to giving advice, making suggestions or comparing experiences. In this sense, co-counselling is truly self-directed and client centred. Courses in co-counselling training, offered by a variety of colleges and extramural departments of universities, are usually of 40 hours in length, run either as a one-week course or as a series of evening classes.

These are some of the practical problems that can occur in counselling and some methods of facing those problems and getting personal support. Sometimes it can be useful to consider some practical questions before setting out to counsel.

- Why has this person come to me?
- Can I help them?
- Have I the necessary knowledge and skills to help?
- What are my beliefs about the nature of the counselling process?
- Why do I want to help this person?
- Do they remind me of anyone I know? This is particularly useful when it comes to the possible development of transference and countertransference. It is important to keep in mind the fact that this person only looks like someone else you know: they are, of course, a separate person!

PROBLEMS AND SUPPORT IN COUNSELLING AND THE HEALTH PROFESSIONAL

All the issues discussed in this chapter apply to a wide range of situations in which the health professional may find themselves, apart from the counselling situation. In other words, the issues of transference and countertransference apply whenever professional and client develop a close relationship. The question of therapeutic distance equally applies to both counselling and all other professional relationships and so does the issue of burnout. In all aspects of health provision, the need for peer support is particularly pertinent. Building a network of support throughout your professional career is a necessity if you are to function effectively and caringly. In order to care effectively for others, we must learn to care for ourselves. In the next chapter, the methods of developing specific counselling skills are described in detail.

11 LEARNING COUNSELLING SKILLS

Three routes are open to the practitioner who wishes to develop a range of counselling skills: working on her own, working as a pair with a colleague or friend or learning in a small group. Each of these routes will be considered in turn and linked to the practical exercises for skills development offered in this book.

Given that this book is all about counselling skills, it might be reasonable to question exactly what we might mean by *skill*. The reader is also referred to Appendix three which identifies the British Association for Counselling's views on counselling training. Barnett (1994) has suggested four criteria for the application of the term 'skill' that are relevant to counselling. Skills involve:

- a situation of some complexity;
- a performance that addresses the situation, is deliberate and is not just a matter of chance;
- an assessment that the performance has met the demands of the situation;
- a sense that the performance was commendable.

WHAT CONSTITUTES AN EFFECTIVE COUNSELLOR

The whole notion of training in counselling raises the question of how we define an effective counsellor. McLeod (1993) suggested the following fairly exhaustive list of areas that might be considered when attempting to assess counselling competence.

- *Interpersonal skills*. Competent counsellors are able to demonstrate appropriate listening, communicating, empathy, presence, awareness of non-verbal communication, sensitivity to voice quality, responsiveness to expressions of emotion, turn taking, structuring of time, use of language.
- *Personal beliefs and attitudes*. Capacity to accept others, belief in the potential for change, awareness of ethical and moral choices. Sensitivity to values held by client and self.
- *Conceptual ability*. Ability to understand and assess the client's problems, to anticipate future consequences of actions, to make sense of immediate process in terms of a wider conceptual scheme, to remember information about the client. Cognitive flexibility. Skill in problem solving.
- *Personal 'soundness'*. Absence of personal needs or irrational beliefs which are destructive to counselling relationships,

self-confidence, capacity to tolerate strong or uncomfortable feelings in relation to clients, secure personal boundaries, ability to be a client. Absence of social prejudice, ethnocentrism and authoritarianism.

- *Mastery of technique*. Knowledge of when and how to carry out specific interventions, ability to access effectiveness of interventions, understanding of rationale behind techniques, possession of a sufficiently wide repertoire of interventions.
- *Ability to understand and work within social systems*. Including awareness of the family and work relationship of the client, the impact of the agency on the client, the capacity to use support networks and supervision. Sensitivity to the social worlds of clients who may be from different gender, ethnic, sexual orientation or age groups.

THE INDIVIDUAL WORKING ALONE

The first consideration is: what knowledge do I need in order to function as an effective counsellor? This may be answered by reference back to the three domains of knowledge covered in Chapter 3: propositional, practical and experiential knowledge. Figure 11.1 identifies some of the types of

Propositional knowledge
• Types of counselling • Maps of the counselling process • Psychological approaches to counselling • Psychology, sociology, philosophy, politics, theology, anthropology
Practical knowledge
• Listening and attending skills • Counselling interventions, including: – being prescriptive – being informative – being confronting – being cathartic – being client centred – being supportive – starting and finishing the session – coping with transference and countertransference – coping with silence – avoiding burnout
Experiential knowledge
• Experience of a wide range of different types of people • Experience of a wide range of human problems • Self-awareness • Spiritual awareness • Cultural awareness • Life experience

Figure 11.1

Aspects of knowledge required for counselling.

knowledge in each of the three domains that the health professional needs to consider.

The person working on her own has a variety of options. She can, for instance, enrol on a counselling skills course. These are offered by colleges and university departments, ranging from one-year certificate courses through two-year diploma courses to Master's degree courses in counselling psychology. Such courses usually cover both the theory and the practice of counselling.

An alternative method is for the person to 'train herself'. This may involve attendance at a number of short counselling workshops in order to identify skilled counselling examples from effective role models, backed up by reading on the topic, reinforced by practice with real clients. Such a solo programme can be helped if the individual can rely on a friend or colleague who is prepared to discuss progress and/or difficult clients. It is also helpful if the person working on her own keeps a journal in which she notes down her progress as a counsellor.

Essential to this method of training is the development of 'conscious use of self' described in Chapter 3. The health professional works at using herself intentionally and notices what she does, both in the counselling relationship and also away from it. Such noticing can bring to attention behaviours and language that are effective and those that are not. Until we notice what we do, we cannot begin to modify or change our behaviour.

WORKING IN PAIRS

Perhaps a more amicable (and less lonely!) way of developing counselling skills is through working with another person. That person can be a member of the family, a friend or a colleague. It is useful if a 'contract' is set up between the two people so that they meet at a regular time each week during which they devote that time to practising counselling skills. In the section on pairs exercises, a whole range of activities are offered which can be worked through by two people. The time spent together can be divided into two and thus one person spends, say, one hour in the role of client and one hour in the role of counsellor. This style of working is not 'role play' as role play suggests acting as a person other than yourself. In the pairs work suggested here, it is recommended that both 'client' and 'counsellor' work on real-life issues during their spell as 'client'. In this way, the self-awareness argued for in previous chapters can be enhanced whilst counselling skills are being developed. Clearly, the subject matter discussed during these sessions must be confidential to the sessions. For this reason, it is often useful if a pair can meet solely for the purpose of practising counselling skills, though this may be difficult to arrange.

At the end of each training session, it is helpful if both parties go through a self and peer evaluation procedure. This involves one person verbalizing her current strengths, weaknesses and things she has learned during the session to her partner. Then the partner offers that person both negative and positive feedback on that person's performance during the training session.

When both self and peer aspects of the evaluation process have been worked through, the two people swap roles and the other person talks through her strengths, weaknesses and things she has learned and then invites feedback from the other person. During the self-evaluation aspects of the process, all that is required of the other person is that she listens. No comments are necessary whilst the other person is evaluating herself – that comes afterwards in the peer evaluation aspect of the process.

Regular meetings between the two partners can be further supplemented by attendance at short training workshops and by further reading on the subject of counselling, counselling psychology and psychotherapy.

WORKING IN A GROUP

The most effective way of training as a counsellor, outside attendance at a formal course of training, is through the setting up of a small training group. This can be made up of colleagues who are interested in developing counselling skills and may be usefully started by the implementation of a one-day workshop to develop basic skills. This can be run at a weekend or, if a one-day slot cannot be found to suit all members of the group, the 'workshop' can be spread over a number of meetings of the group.

An alternative to the self-help or 'do-it-yourself' group is the more formal educational group, set up by the educational body responsible for training staff in the health organization. Both groups can use the outline programme described below for running a counselling skills workshop.

Figure 11.2 offers a sample programme outline for such a workshop. It may be given to participants before the workshop or it may be allowed to 'unfold' as the workshop develops. The advantage of giving it out prior to the workshop is that it offers minimal but essential structure. Many people attending workshops seem to prefer and anticipate structure and this programme can satisfy that need. On the other hand, the advantage of allowing the programme to 'unfold' is that it ensures that the workshop is a dynamic and organic process that responds to the needs and wants of the participants as they arise. In the end, the structure is governed by the personal preference of the person setting up the workshop and, perhaps, their previous experience in running groups of this sort.

Setting the learning climate

This is the first stage of the counselling skills workshop. It involves at least the following activities:

- introductions;
- expectations;
- rationale for the workshop.

The 'introductions' aspect involves helping group members to get to know each other and to remember each other's names. A variety of 'icebreakers' are described in the literature which some people prefer to use as a means

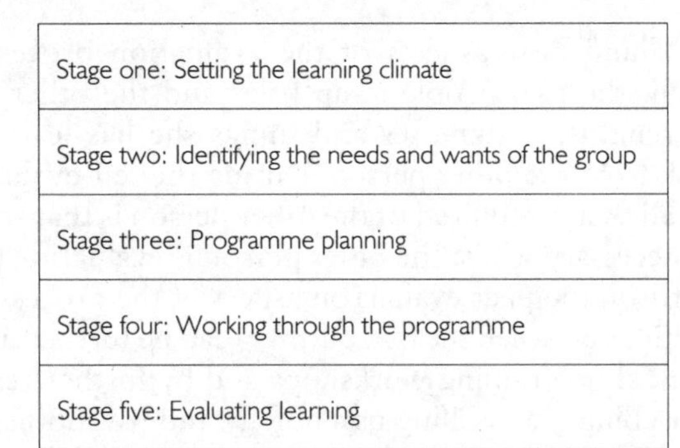

Figure 11.2

Stages in a counselling skills workshop.

of starting the workshop (Heron, 1973; Brandes and Philips, 1984; Burnard, 1985). Three examples of such icebreakers are as follows.

Icebreaker one

Group members stand up and move around the room. At a signal from the group leader, they stop and pair off with their nearest colleague. The pairs then spend a few minutes sharing their thoughts on one of the following:

- childhood memories;
- interests away from work;
- personal interests in counselling.

After a few minutes, the leader suggests that the group move on and pair up with other people. They then spend a few minutes in those pairs discussing similar issues.

Icebreaker two

Group members, in turn, recall three positive and formative experiences from their lives and share those experiences with the rest of the group.

Icebreaker three

The group leader asks each person in turn to imagine that they are one of the following objects: a book, a piece of music or a film. The group member is then asked to describe herself as though she was that object. Thus, the leader asks one of the following questions.

- If you were a book, what book would you be? Describe yourself as that book.
- If you were a piece of music, what piece would you be? Describe yourself as that piece of music.
- If you were a film, what film would you be? Describe yourself as that film.

Again, the use of such icebreakers may be a question of personal preference. Some group leaders (and workshop participants) may find them difficult to use or to take part in. They seem to suit the more extroverted (and possibly younger) participants. However, they can allow people to unwind a little and thus prepare for some of the pairs and group activities described below.

A quieter method of introducing a counselling skills workshop is to invite each member in turn to identify the following things about themselves:

- their name;
- their present job;
- their background;
- their interests away from work.

After they have disclosed themselves to the group in this way, each member is invited to repeat his or her name slowly and in turn. This can be repeated two or three times until all members are sure of each other's names.

Following these introductory activities, group members may be invited to pair off and discuss their expectations about the coming workshop and about future group meetings. Such expectations may include both negative and positive things. The point here is that all members be given the opportunity to explore how they feel about the coming time together and are able to share fantasies, hopes and anxieties. Following this ten-minute exercise, the group may be invited to reform and those expectations are discussed. It is usually helpful to discuss negative expectations first, followed by the positive.

Once expectations have been fully explored (a process that may take between 30 minutes and one hour), the group leader may offer a rationale for the workshop, which will include the leader's explanation of her reasons for organizing the workshop in this manner and what the workshop is intended to be about. It may also include negotiation with the group of basic ground rules for the workshop. These may cover such things as:

- rules about smoking;
- issues relating to coffee, tea and meal breaks;
- a 'proposal' clause;
- a 'voluntary' clause.

A proposal clause means that any member of the group may propose changes to the format or structure of the group at any time. It may also be used to encourage group members to take responsibility for ensuring that they get what they want from the workshop. If they are not, then they should feel free to propose a change of activity.

A voluntary clause stresses the idea that participation in any aspect of the workshop or the group meetings is voluntary. As all counselling workshops are organized for adults, its seems reasonable to assume that they will decide, as individuals, what does and what does not enhance their learning.

It seems reasonable, too, that no part of the workshop should be compulsory.

Identifying the needs/wants of the group

This next process is one that naturally leads into programme planning. The group is invited to form into small groups of three and four. Each group 'brainstorms' onto a large sheet of paper the things that they require from the workshop. Such requirements may be particular skills, various sorts of knowledge or some sort of personal development. It is useful, too, at this stage to identify any particular resources in the group. Some group members may have particular counselling exercises that they feel others may benefit from. Others may have particular knowledge about counselling theory. Figure 11.3 demonstrates the layout of the sheet for use in the small group.

When the small groups have had sufficient time to complete the brainstorming exercise, they are invited to prioritize their list of needs and wants. Once this is completed, a feedback session will ensure that group priorities are identified and offers made by individuals are recognized.

Out of the previous activity develops the programme for the counselling workshop. This stage involves negotiating the timing of activities required by the group. It also involves fitting in those activities with any preplanned activities that the leader has brought to the workshop. It is useful, at this stage, to offer group members a skeleton programme plan which contains various 'blanks' into which go the activities identified in the above exercise. An example of a typical programme is offered in Figure 11.4. The 'sessions' referred to in the outline programme are times when the exercises that follow in this book may be used to develop specific counselling skills. Alternatively, those sessions can be made up of exercises offered by other group members.

NEEDS AND WANTS Identify here anything that you need to gain from this counselling workshop. You can list theories, skills – anything.	OFFERS Identify here anything you are prepared to share with the group (skills, knowledge, activities, etc.)

Figure 11.3

Layout for a brainstorming exercise

9.00–10.00 Introductions
10.00–10.30 Coffee
10.30–12.00 Identification of needs/wants and programme planning
12.00–1.00 First skills training session
1.00–2.00 Lunch
2.00–3.00 Second skills training session
3.00–3.15 Tea
3.15–4.15 Third skills training session
4.15–5.00 Evaluation

Figure 11.4

Example of a 'skeleton' counselling skills workshop programme.

Working through the programme

Once the programme has been negotiated, all that remains is for the sessions to be undertaken as planned. Given that the workshop and subsequent group meetings are about counselling, it is useful if the experiential learning cycle is observed through each session (Kolb, 1984; Burnard, 1985). Experiential learning is learning through doing, through immediate personal experience. A modification of the cycle is demonstrated in Figure 11.5.

First, a brief theory input is offered to the group. This may be on a particular aspect of counselling or a description of a counselling skill. It is helpful, too, if the group can see some examples of 'excellent practice' in counselling as a basis for their own counselling skills. Such examples may be shown on video or film or skilled practitioners may be invited to demonstrate counselling practice 'live'. This use of exemplars is particularly helpful in the early stages of counselling skills workshops and counselling skills development. Once group members have established a basic range of their own skills, the exemplars can be dropped.

Then an activity is undertaken by the group, either as a whole or with the group split into pairs, in order to practise a particular counselling skill.

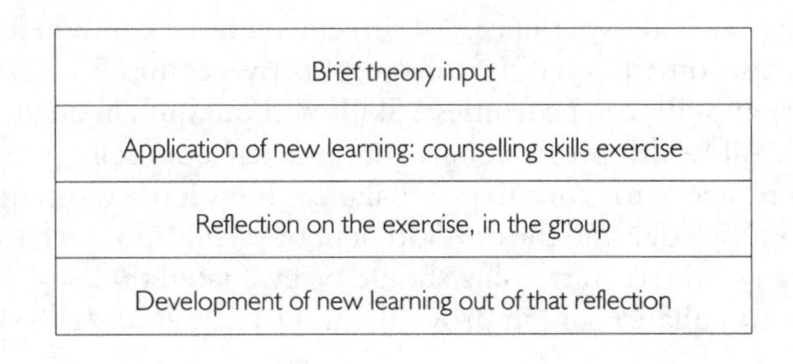

Brief theory input
Application of new learning: counselling skills exercise
Reflection on the exercise, in the group
Development of new learning out of that reflection

Figure 11.5

The experiential learning cycle applied to counselling skills development.

When the activity has finished (and details of how to set up and run those activities are offered with each exercise in the pages that follow), group members are invited to reflect on the experience and draw new learning from it. That learning is then applied and implications for future behaviour are discussed. It is vital that all new learning is carried over from the workshop situation to the 'real' situation with clients; new counselling skills have to be practised as soon as possible away from the workshop to maximize the efficacy of the activity.

Evaluating learning

At the end of the workshop, the group needs to evaluate their learning. This can be done formally, through the use of a written evaluative questionnaire (Clift and Imrie, 1981; Patton, 1982) prepared prior to the workshop. Alternatively, it can be carried out through the process of self and peer evaluation, which involves the following stages:

- identification of criteria for evaluation;
- group members silently evaluating themselves using those criteria;
- group members, in turn, verbalizing their evaluation to the group;
- group members, in turn, inviting feedback from the group on their own performance during the workshop.

This process may be followed by a closing 'round' of what each group member liked least about the workshop followed by a round of what each member liked most. This rounds off the proceedings and reinforces themes and learning gained within the workshop.

This format for running a one-day workshop can be adapted for use at subsequent meetings of the counselling skills learning group. At each meeting, a short period can be used to 'warm up' the group, using icebreakers or similar activities. Then the group members can decide on what they want to achieve during the meeting. A series of counselling skills exercises can be used, drawn from this book or from others (see, for example, Lewis and Streitfield, 1971; Heron, 1973; Pfeiffer and Jones, 1974; Wilkinson and Canter, 1982; Egan, 1986). After each exercise, a reflective period can allow consideration of how the new skill may be implemented in the 'real' situation. Finally, the meeting can close with an evaluation activity.

These, then, are three approaches to counselling skills training that can be used separately or in combination. All three emphasize the need for practice and for practical experience. All three need to be combined with constant reflection on the qualities of the effective counsellor. Counselling without certain skills can be fruitless. Skills without human qualities will be mechanical. All health professionals who practise counselling as an aspect of their job need to consider a balance between counselling skills, up-to-date knowledge and the development of caring approach to people.

Clearly, any courses of training should be evaluated thoroughly in order to continue to enhance and improve them. Dryden *et al.* (1995) list what might be reviewed during an internal audit of a counselling course. They recommend that the following information might be sought.

- Number of applications received, applicants interviewed, places offered and places accepted.
- Number of students in each cohort or year group, dropouts and reasons for leaving.
- Number of students passing the course.
- Information on employment changes of students as a result of taking the course.
- Student feedback and evaluation including summary of comments.
- External examiner's report or evaluation.
- Staff response to critical feedback from students or external examiner.
- Changes or solutions to problems during the year.
- Proposed developments or improvements for future courses.
- Staff professional and academic development activities.
- Extraordinary achievements of the course or students.
- Organizational problems beyond the responsibility of the staff team.

LEARNING COUNSELLING SKILLS AND THE HEALTH PROFESSIONAL

As we have noted throughout this book, the skills described as 'counselling skills' also have wider application outside the counselling relationship and can be used to enhance professional practice in any branch of the caring and health professions. The format for organizing the learning of counselling skills, described in this chapter, can also be adapted for learning or developing a whole range of interpersonal skills related to health care, including interviewing, stress management, self-awareness, assertiveness, assessment and evaluation.

12 COUNSELLING SKILLS EXERCISES

In the previous chapter, we discussed how to develop counselling skills, working alone, in pairs or in a small group. This chapter offers a range of counselling skills exercises and activities. The first group is for the individual working on her own, the second group is pairs activities and the third is group activities. The second and third group may be used in combination by a group of colleagues working together to enhance their counselling skills. Each exercise should be worked through slowly with plenty of time allowed for 'processing' or discussing the activity afterwards.

As we noted in the last chapter, a useful format for a counselling skills training session is as follows.

- Identification of how the group wants to spend the time.
- A theory input and some examples of good counselling practice, either 'live' or shown on video or film.
- Using a variety of exercises to develop counselling skills.
- Evaluation activities.

Built into each of the pairs and group exercises are the means to evaluate learning at the end of each activity. It is recommended that the evaluation procedure is followed fairly closely so that the maximum amount of learning may be gained from each exercise. The list of exercises below is not exhaustive and many more may be gleaned from the literature listed in the bibliography. Many exercises may also be developed by group members themselves.

The pairs format is particularly useful. In this, the group breaks into pairs, each member of which spends some time in the roles of 'counsellor' and of 'client'. After a period of practising specific counselling skills, the partners swap roles. This format can be used on a regular basis for practising counselling and may be combined with receiving feedback on skills development from the partner.

All the work carried out individually, in pairs or in a group must be followed up quickly by real-life experience. Thus the counsellor must learn to develop the 'conscious use of self' referred to throughout this book. In this way, the health professional can make full use of any learning gained by putting it into practice, in real counselling situations. Like all skills, counselling skills must be reinforced if they are to become a regular part of the person's repertoire of behaviour.

ACTIVITIES Exercises for the person working alone

Exercise No. 1

Aim of the Exercise
To clarify beliefs and values, prior to undertaking counselling.

Process of the Exercise
Write out in a free style a paper which expresses your current set of values and beliefs about human beings, counselling and about yourself. Do not try to make the paper 'academic' in any way and do not worry about style or presentation. Once you have written the paper, consider whether or not it highlights any ambiguities or contradictions in your construing of the world. If so, consider whether or not you will attempt to resolve those contradictions. Consider, also, ways in which your beliefs and values affect your work and your attitude towards counselling. You may or may not choose to show the paper to someone else and have them comment on it.

Exercise No. 2

Aim of the Exercise
To consider aspects of yourself and your work that will help or hinder your counselling.

Process of the Exercise
'Brainstorm' onto a sheet of paper all those aspects of yourself and your work that you bring to your counselling work. Include in your list those aspects of yourself and your work that you anticipate will cause difficulties. Allow yourself to think and write quickly. Once the list has become fairly lengthy, organize it into 'pluses' and 'minuses'. Consider the degree to which one list is longer than the other and the implications of that. Consider also what you intend to do about the 'minuses'.

Exercise No. 3

Aim of the Exercise
To enable a continuous means of personal evaluation to be maintained.

Process of the Exercise
Keep a journal from the point of taking up counselling. Use the following headings to order the journal:

- recent skills developed;
- recent problems encountered and problem-solving methods used;
- new references to books and journals noted;
- aspects of personal growth.

Journals may usefully be kept by all members of a group working together on developing counselling skills. At each meeting of the group, time can be set aside to discuss journal entries.

Exercise No. 4

Aim of the Exercise
To develop 'conscious use of self'.

Process of the Exercise
Set aside a time each day when you notice what you do and how you do it. Notice patterns of behaviour, speech, proximity to others, use of touch, hand and arm gestures, social skills and so on. Try out new behaviour and new counselling skills as they develop. Allow this time to develop and lengthen until you become more aware of how you react and interact.

Exercise No. 5

Aim of the Exercise
To develop the ability to 'notice'.

Process of the Exercise
Noticing (sometimes called 'staying awake' or 'conscious awareness') involves setting aside time each day to notice everything that is going on around you. Notice sounds, smells, colours, activity, objects and so on. Allow this period of noticing to develop and lengthen. Use the activity particularly when you are with other people.

Exercise No. 6

Aim of the Exercise
To develop observational skills, 'conscious use of self' and the ability to 'notice'.

Process of the Exercise
Spend 20 minutes each evening sitting in the same place and at the same time. Allow your attention to focus only on those things that you see, hear, smell or feel outside yourself. Do not attempt to evaluate what comes in through your senses, but only notice them. Regular use of this activity (akin to certain types of meditation) will improve your ability to keep your attention 'out' and will improve your observational skills.

Exercise No. 7

Aim of the Exercise
To experience physical changes in the body, to become more aware of the body and to physically relax.

Process of the Exercise
Find a quiet, warm place in which you can lie down for about half an hour, undisturbed. Once you have lain down, take three deep breaths. Then allow your attention to focus on the muscles in your face. Let them relax. Then focus your attention on the muscles in your shoulders and upper arms. Let them relax. Focus your attention on the muscles in your lower arms and hands. Stretch out your fingers. Then let your arms relax. Then put your attention on the muscles in your chest and stomach. Let those muscles relax. Then focus on the muscles in your legs and stretch your feet forward. Then let all the muscles in your legs relax. Then notice how all the muscles in your body are relaxed. Allow yourself to notice what it feels like to be relaxed. Notice, too, parts of the body that you find difficult to relax. After about ten minutes, stretch gently, allow yourself to sit up and then slowly stand up. Notice the difference in the way you feel before and after the activity.

This exercise may also be used as a stress reduction activity with clients who find it difficult to relax. It can also be dictated onto a tape for use as a means of deep relaxation.

Exercise No. 8

Aim of the Exercise
To identify personal strengths and weaknesses in terms of counselling interventions.

Process of the Exercise
Consider Heron's (1986) six-category intervention analysis:

- *Prescriptive interventions:* giving advice, offering suggestions.
- *Informative interventions:* offering information.
- *Confronting interventions:* challenging.
- *Cathartic interventions:* helping the client to express emotion.
- *Catalytic interventions:* 'drawing out' the client.
- *Supportive interventions:* encouraging, validating the client.

Identify the two categories that you feel you are least skilled in using at the moment. Then consider the two categories that you are most skilled in using. Consider the implications of your assessment and think of ways in which you can enhance your deficiencies.

Exercise No. 9

Aim of the Exercise
To plan future objectives.

Process of the Exercise
Write down a list of the counselling skills or aspects of counselling that you need to improve upon. Make each of them a specific, behavioural objective and ones that are attainable. Then determine how you will meet those objectives.

ACTIVITIES Exercises for people working in pairs

Exercise No. 10

Aim of the Exercise
To experience problems associated with listening.

Equipment Required/Environmental Considerations
The pair should sit facing each other in chairs of equal height. It is helpful if the room is comfortably warm and free from distractions and interruptions.

Process of the Exercise
The pair divide themselves into A and B. A talks to B on any subject for four minutes and B does not listen! After the four minutes, roles are reversed and B talks to A, who does not listen! After the second round, the pair discuss the activity.

Evaluation Procedure
At the end of the exercise each person should report to the other what they disliked and what they liked about the activity. They may also comment on what they will be able to carry over from it into the 'real' counselling situation.

Exercise No. 11

Aim of the Exercise
To experience problems with the non-verbal aspects of listening.

Equipment Required/Environmental Considerations
The pair should sit facing each other in chairs of equal height. It is helpful if the room is comfortably warm and free from distractions and interruptions.

Process of the Exercise
The pair divide themselves into A and B. A talks to B for four minutes about any topic and B listens but contradicts the first four aspects of the SOLER behaviours identified by Egan (1986). Thus, B does not sit squarely in relation to A. She folds her arms and her legs. She leans away from her partner and makes no eye contact with her. After four minutes, roles are reversed and B talks to A, while A listens but offers contradictory behaviours. After the second four minutes, the pair discuss the exercise.

Evaluation Procedure
At the end of the exercise each person should report to the other what they disliked and what they liked about the activity. They may also

comment on what they will be able to carry over from it into the 'real' counselling situation.

Exercise No. 12

Aim of the Exercise

To experience effective listening and to enhance listening skills.

Equipment Required/Environmental Considerations

The pair should sit facing each other in chairs of equal height. It is helpful if the room is comfortably warm and free from distractions and interruptions.

Process of the Exercise

The pair divide themselves into A and B. A talks to B for four minutes about any topic and B listens, observing the SOLER behaviours. Thus, she sits squarely in an open position. She leans slightly towards her partner and maintains good eye contact. She also relaxes and does nothing but listen. It is important that this is not a conversation but a listening exercise! After four minutes, roles are reversed and B talks to A, who listens appropriately. After the second four minutes the pair discuss the exercise and compare it with the previous two.

Evaluation Procedure

At the end of the exercise each person should report to the other what they disliked and what they liked about the activity. They may also comment on what they will be able to carry over from it into the 'real' counselling situation.

Exercise No. 13

Aim of the Exercise

To practise effective listening and to evaluate the effectiveness of the listening.

Equipment Required/Environmental Considerations

The pair should sit facing each other in chairs of equal height. It is helpful if the room is comfortably warm and free from distractions and interruptions.

Process of the Exercise

The pair divide themselves into A and B. A talks to B for four minutes on any topic. B listens and periodically 'recaps' on what A has said, to A's satisfaction. After four minutes, roles are reversed and B talks to A, who listens and periodically recaps. After a further four minutes, the pair discuss the exercise.

Evaluation Procedure

At the end of the exercise each person should report to the other what they disliked and what they liked about the activity. They may also comment on what they will be able to carry over from it into the 'real' counselling situation.

Exercise No. 14

Aim of the Exercise

To discriminate between open and closed questions.

Equipment Required/Environmental Considerations

The pair should sit facing each other in chairs of equal height. It is helpful if the room is comfortably warm and free from distractions and interruptions. A pencil and paper are needed for this activity.

Process of the Exercise

Both partners jot down the following sequence O,O,C,C,O,C,O,C. Then the pair divide themselves into A and B. A then asks questions of B on any of the following topics: current issues at work, recent holidays, the current political situation. The questions are asked in the sequence noted above (i.e. 'open question, open question, closed question, closed question' and so on) until all the above questions have been asked. Then the pair swap roles and B asks questions of A, in that sequence and on one of those topics.

Evaluation Procedure

At the end of the exercise each person should report to the other what they disliked and what they liked about the activity. They may also comment on what they will be able to carry over from it into the 'real' counselling situation.

Exercise No. 15

Aim of the Exercise

To practise funnelling in questioning.

Equipment Required/Environmental Considerations

The pair should sit facing each other in chairs of equal height. It is helpful if the room is comfortably warm and free from distractions and interruptions.

Process of the Exercise

The pair divide themselves into A and B. A then asks questions of B on any subject they wish, starting with a very broad open question and slowly allowing the questions to become more specific and focused. After four minutes, the pair swap roles and B asks questions of A, moving from the general to the particular.

Evaluation Procedure
At the end of the exercise each person should report to the other what they disliked and what they liked about the activity. They may also comment on what they will be able to carry over from it into the 'real' counselling situation.

Exercise No. 16

Aim of the Exercise
To practise 'reflection' and 'selective reflection'.

Equipment Required/Environmental Considerations
The pair should sit facing each other in chairs of equal height. It is helpful if the room is comfortably warm and free from distractions and interruptions.

Process of the Exercise
The pair divide themselves into A and B. A talks to B about any subject and A uses only reflection or selective reflection to encourage her to continue. This should be continued for about six minutes. After six minutes, roles are reversed and B talks to A who uses only reflection or selective reflection as a response. For details of these two techniques, see page 124.

Evaluation Procedure
At the end of the exercise each person should report to the other what they disliked and what they liked about the activity. They may also comment on what they will be able to carry over from it into the 'real' counselling situation.

Exercise No. 17

Aim of the Exercise
To practise a range of client centred counselling skills.

Equipment Required/Environmental Considerations
The pair should sit facing each other in chairs of equal height. It is helpful if the room is comfortably warm and free from distractions and interruptions.

Process of the Exercise
The pair divide themselves into A and B. A then begins to 'counsel' B but restricts herself to the following types of interventions:

- open or closed questions;
- reflections or selective reflections;
- checking for understanding;
- empathy-building statements.

The counselling session should continue for at least ten minutes, then change roles for a further ten minutes. There should be no sense of play acting or role playing about the exercise. Both partners should counsel on 'real' issues and thus develop realistic skills. This exercise, like the previous one, is very difficult because both parties are 'in the know'!

Evaluation Procedure
At the end of the exercise each person should report to the other what they disliked and what they liked about the activity. They may also comment on what they will be able to carry over from it into the 'real' counselling situation.

Exercise No. 18

Aim of the Exercise
To experience being asked a wide range of questions.

Equipment Required/Environmental Considerations
The pair should sit facing each other in chairs of equal height. It is helpful if the room is comfortably warm and free from distractions and interruptions.

Process of the Exercise
The pair divide themselves into A and B. A then asks a wide range of questions, on any topic at all, for five minutes and B does not respond to them or answer them! After five minutes, roles are reversed and B asks questions of A, who does not respond to them. It is important for both partners to notice how they feel about asking and being asked very personal questions.

Evaluation Procedure
At the end of the exercise each person should report to the other what they disliked and what they liked about the activity. They may also comment on what they will be able to carry over from it into the 'real' counselling situation.

Exercise No. 19

Aim of the Exercise
To notice the difference between being asked questions and making statements.

Equipment Required/Environmental Considerations
The pair should sit facing each other in chairs of equal height. It is helpful if the room is comfortably warm and free from distractions and interruptions.

Process of the Exercise
The pair divide themselves into A and B. A makes a series of statements, on any topic, to B for five minutes. B listens to the statements but does not respond to them. After five minutes, roles are reversed and B makes a series of statements to A who only listens. Afterwards, the pair discuss the perceived differences between how this exercise felt and how the previous one felt. They discuss, also, the relative merits of questions and statements with regard to counselling.

Evaluation Procedure
At the end of the exercise each person should report to the other what they disliked and what they liked about the activity. They may also comment on what they will be able to carry over from it into the 'real' counselling situation.

Exercise No. 20

Aim of the Exercise
To explore personal history.

Equipment Required/Environmental Considerations:
The pair should sit facing each other in chairs of equal height. It is helpful if the room is comfortably warm and free from distractions and interruptions.

Process of the Exercise
The pair divide themselves into A and B. A talks to B for ten minutes and reviews her life history to date. Any aspects may be included or left out but some sort of chronological order should be aimed at. After ten minutes, roles are reversed and B reviews her biography to date, while A listens but does not comment.

Evaluation Procedure
At the end of the exercise each person should report to the other what they disliked and what they liked about the activity. They may also comment on what they will be able to carry over from it into the 'real' counselling situation.

Exercise No. 21

Aim of the Exercise
To explore 'free association'.

Equipment Required/Environmental Considerations
The pair should sit facing each other in chairs of equal height. It is helpful if the room is comfortably warm and free from distractions and interruptions.

Process of the Exercise
The pair divide themselves into A and B. A verbalizes whatever comes into her head, whilst B sits and listens only. Everything possible should be verbalized but A should note the things that she does not verbalize! This process continues for three minutes when the pair swap roles and B attempts 'free association' accompanied by A's attention and listening. Afterwards the pair discuss the implications of the activity for themselves and for their counselling practice.

Evaluation Procedure
At the end of the exercise each person should report to the other what they disliked and what they liked about the activity. They may also comment on what they will be able to carry over from it into the 'real' counselling situation.

Exercise No. 22

Aim of the Exercise
To self evaluate.

Equipment Required/Environmental Considerations
The pair should sit facing each other in chairs of equal height. It is helpful if the room is comfortably warm and free from distractions and interruptions.

Process of the Exercise
The pair divide themselves into A and B. A then considers and verbalizes all the positive and negative aspects of her counselling practice to date. Negative considerations should be made first. When A has finished, B goes through the same process. Afterwards, the pair consider the implications of their evaluations for their counselling practice.

Evaluation Procedure
At the end of the exercise each person should report to the other what they disliked and what they liked about the activity. They may also comment on what they will be able to carry over from it into the 'real' counselling situation.

Exercise No. 23

Aim of the Exercise
To receive feedback on counselling skills.

Equipment Required/Environmental Considerations
The pair should sit facing each other in chairs of equal height. It is helpful if the room is comfortably warm and free from distractions and interruptions.

Process of the Exercise
The pair divide themselves into A and B. A then offers B both positive and negative feedback as to how she perceives the other's counselling skills. Negative comments should be made first. Then B offers A feedback on her counselling skills. Afterwards both partners consider the implications of this feedback for their counselling practice and compare it with their own self-evaluation.

Evaluation Procedure
At the end of the exercise each person should report to the other what they disliked and what they liked about the activity. They may also comment on what they will be able to carry over from it into the 'real' counselling situation.

ACTIVITIES Exercises for people working in groups

Exercise No. 24

Aim of the Exercise
To increase the listening and attending skills of group members

Number of Participants
Any number between five and 20.

Time Required
Between 1 and 1½ hours.

Equipment Required / Environmental Considerations
The group should sit in chairs of equal height and in a circle. It is helpful if the room is comfortably warm and does not contain too many distractions.

Process of the Exercise
The group holds a discussion on any topic. One ground rule applies throughout the exercise: once the first person has spoken, before anyone else contributes to the discussion, they must first summarize what the person before them has said, to that person's satisfaction! After half an hour, the group discusses the activity.

Evaluation Procedure
Learning from the exercise is evaluated by two 'rounds'. First, each person in turn says what she did not like about the exercise. Then, each person in turn says what she did like about the activity. A third round can be used to establish how each person will use the learning gained in the future.

Variations on the Exercise
1 The facilitator chooses a topic for discussion, e.g.:

- qualities of the effective counsellor;
- how we can become better counsellors;
- how is this group developing.

2 The larger group can break into small groups of four or five to carry out the exercise and then have a plenary session back in the larger group.

Exercise No. 25

Aim of the Exercise
To practise asking questions in a group and to experience being asked questions.

Number of Participants
Any number between five and 20.

Time Required
Between 1 and $1\frac{1}{2}$ hours.

Equipment Required / Environmental Considerations
The group should sit in chairs of equal height and in a circle. It is helpful if the room is comfortably warm and does not contain too many distractions.

Process of the Exercise
Each person in turn spends five minutes in the 'hot seat'. When occupying the hot seat, they may be asked questions on any subject by any member of the group. If they wish not to answer a particular question, they may say 'pass'. At the end of the five minutes the person nominates the next person to occupy it, until all members of the group have had a five-minute turn.

Procedure
Learning from the exercise is evaluated by two 'rounds'. First, each person in turn says what she did not like about the exercise. Then, each person in turn says what she did like about the activity. A third round can be used to establish how each person will use the learning gained in the future.

Variations on the Exercise
1 The time in the 'hot seat' may be varied from two to ten minutes depending upon the size of the group and the time available.
2 A large group may be split up into smaller groups.
3 With a group in which members know each other very well, the 'pass' facility may be abandoned!

Exercise No. 26

Aim of the Exercise
To experience clear communication within the group.

Number of Participants
Any number between five and 20.

Time Required
Between 1 and $1\frac{1}{2}$ hours.

Equipment Required / Environmental Considerations
The group should sit in chairs of equal height and in a circle. It is helpful if the room is comfortably warm and does not contain too many distractions.

Process of the Exercise
The group hold a discussion on any topic and observe the following ground rules:

- speak directly, using 'I' rather than 'you', 'we' or 'one';
- speak directly to others, using the first person;
- stay in the present;
- avoid theorizing about what is going on in the group.

Either the facilitator acts as guardian of the ground rules or the group monitors itself.

Evaluation Procedure
Learning from the exercise is evaluated by two 'rounds'. First, each person in turn says what she did not like about the exercise. Then, each person in turn says what she did like about the activity. A third round can be used to establish how each person will use the learning gained in the future.

Variations on the Exercise
1 No topic is chosen by or for the group: the material for discussion evolves out of what is happening in the 'here and now'.

Exercise No. 27

Aim of the Exercise
To experience participation in a 'leaderless' group and to consider the dynamics of such an activity.

Number of Participants
Any number between five and 20.

Time Required
Between 1 and 1½ hours.

Equipment Required / Environmental Considerations
The group should sit in chairs of equal height and in a circle. It is helpful if the room is comfortably warm and does not contain too many distractions. An object to use as a 'conch' is required.

Process of the Exercise
The group have a discussion on any topic. In order to speak, however, they must be in possession of the 'conch'; an object which signifies that, at that moment, the person holding it is leading the group. Other people who wish to speak must non-verbally negotiate for possession of the conch. After about half an hour, the group drop the 'conch' rule and freely discuss the activity.

Evaluation Procedure
Learning from the exercise is evaluated by two 'rounds'. First, each person in turn says what she did not like about the exercise. Then, each person in

turn says what she did like about the activity. A third round can be used to establish how each person will use the learning gained in the future.

Variations on the Exercise

1 The facilitator chooses a topic for the group to discuss.
2 A rule may be introduced whereby each person may only make one statement when in possession of the 'conch'.

Exercise No. 28

Aim of the Exercise

To practise using client-centred counselling interventions in a group.

Number of Participants

Any number between five and 20.

Time Required

Between 1 and 1½ hours.

Equipment Required / Environmental Considerations

The group should sit in chairs of equal height and in a circle. It is helpful if the room is comfortably warm and does not contain too many distractions.

Process of the Exercise

The group members are only allowed to:

- ask questions of each other;
- practise reflections;
- offer empathy-building statements;
- check for understanding of each other.

After half an hour, the group discusses the exercise, having dropped the rule about types of interventions.

Evaluation Procedure

Learning from the exercise is evaluated by two 'rounds'. First, each person in turn says what she did not like about the exercise. Then, each person in turn says what she did like about the activity. A third round can be used to establish how each person will use the learning gained in the future.

Variations on the Exercise

1 One group member is invited to facilitate a general discussion with the group, using only: a) questions, b) reflections, c) empathy-building statements or d) checking for understanding. Afterwards, the group offers that person feedback on her performance.
2 Group members, in turn, facilitate a discussion using only the above types of interventions, for periods of ten minutes each.

Exercise No. 29

Aim of the Exercise
To explore silence in a group context.

Number of Participants
Any number between five and 20.

Time Required
Between 1 and 1½ hours.

Equipment Required / Environmental Considerations
The group should sit in chairs of equal height and in a circle. It is helpful if the room is comfortably warm and does not contain too many distractions.

Process of the Exercise
The group facilitator suggests to the group that they sit in total silence for a period of five minutes. When the five minutes is over, the group discusses the experience.

Evaluation Procedure
Learning from the exercise is evaluated by two 'rounds'. First, each person in turn says what she did not like about the exercise. Then, each person in turn says what she did like about the activity. A third round can be used to establish how each person will use the learning gained in the future.

Variations on the Exercise
The group may sit in silence with their eyes closed.

Exercise No. 30

Aim of the Exercise
To explore a variety of facets of counselling.

Number of Participants
Any number between five and 20.

Time Required
Between 1 and 1½ hours.

Equipment Required / Environmental Considerations
The group should sit in chairs of equal height and in a circle. It is helpful if the room is comfortably warm and does not contain too many distractions. A large sheet of paper or a black or white board is required for this activity.

Process of the Exercise

The group carries out a 'brainstorming' activity. One member of the group acts as 'scribe' and jots down on a large sheet of paper or a black/white board all comments from the group on one of the following topics. No contributions are discarded and group members are encouraged to call out any associations they make with the topic

- qualities of an effective counsellor;
- problems/difficulties of this group;
- activities for improving counselling skills;
- qualities of the ineffective counsellor;
- skills required for effective counselling;
- problems that health professionals are likely to encounter in counselling.

Evaluation Procedure

Learning from the exercise is evaluated by two 'rounds'. First, each person in turn says what she did not like about the exercise. Then, each person in turn says what she did like about the activity. A third round can be used to establish how each person will use the learning gained in the future.

Exercise No. 31

Aim of the Exercise

To receive feedback from other group members.

Number of Participants

Any number between five and 20.

Time Required

Between 1 and 1½ hours.

Equipment Required / Environmental Considerations

The group should sit in chairs of equal height and in a circle. It is helpful if the room is comfortably warm and does not contain too many distractions.

Process of the Exercise

Each member of the group in turn listens to other members of the group offering her positive feedback, i.e. things they like about that person. The feedback is given in the form of a 'round', with each person in turn offering feedback until every group member has spoken. The group member receiving feedback is not allowed to 'respond' to the comments but must listen in silence!

Evaluation Procedure

Learning from the exercise is evaluated by two 'rounds'. First, each person in turn says what she did not like about the exercise. Then, each person in turn says what she did like about the activity. A third round can be used to establish how each person will use the learning gained in the future.

Variations on the Exercise

1 With a group where members know each other very well, a round of negative feedback may be offered to each group member, if they require it. This activity should be handled with care!

Exercise No. 32

Aim of the Exercise

To carry out a peer and group evaluation.

Number of Participants

Any number between five and 20.

Time Required

Between 1 and 1½ hours.

Equipment Required / Environmental Considerations

The group should sit in chairs of equal height and in a circle. It is helpful if the room is comfortably warm and does not contain too many distractions.

Process of the Exercise

The group identifies six criteria for evaluating members of the group, e.g.:

- contribution to activities;
- self-disclosure;
- contribution of new ideas to the group, etc., etc.

Then each group member silently jots down her own evaluation of herself under these six headings. When all members have finished, each reads out their notes to the rest of the group and invites feedback from other group members on those six criteria. The process is repeated until all group members have both verbalized their evaluation and received feedback from other group members.

Evaluation Procedure

Learning from the exercise is evaluated by two 'rounds'. First, each person in turn says what she did not like about the exercise. Then, each person in turn says what she did like about the activity. A third round can be used to establish how each person will use the learning gained in the future.

Variations on the Exercise

The feedback from the group may be offered systematically: each group member in turn, working round the group, offers the individual feedback on her performance.

Exercise No. 33

Aim of the Exercise
To explore a spontaneous and leaderless group activity the 'Quaker' group.

Number of Participants
Any number between five and 20.

Time Required
Between 1 and 1½ hours.

Equipment Required / Environmental Considerations
The group should sit in chairs of equal height and in a circle. It is helpful if the room is comfortably warm and does not contain too many distractions.

Process of the Exercise
The group has no topic for discussion and no leader. Group members are encouraged to verbalize what they are feeling and thinking as those thoughts and feeling occur but there is no obligation for anyone else to respond to the statements offered. The group may fall into silence at times and at others be very noisy! The group exercise should be allowed to run for at least three-quarters of an hour. After that period, group members can freely discuss how it felt to take part in the activity.

Evaluation Procedure
Learning from the exercise is evaluated by two 'rounds'. First, each person in turn says what she did not like about the exercise. Then, each person in turn says what she did like about the activity. A third round can be used to establish how each person will use the learning gained in the future.

Variations on the Exercise
A topic may be chosen for the group to consider, but no direction is offered by the group facilitator and group members make statements about the topic as and when they choose.

COUNSELLING SKILLS AND THE HEALTH PROFESSIONAL

These are a range of counselling skills exercises that have been used by the writer in a variety of contexts to help in the development of counselling and interpersonal skills. They can be modified and adapted to suit the specific needs of particular groups of health professionals. Often, too, as we have noted, the best exercises are those that you devise yourself: the group that learns to identify its particular needs and then develops exercises to explore a particular skill can quickly become an autonomous learning group.

Learning to practise as a counsellor can be an exciting and challenging process. It is hoped that this book has offered some signposts to directions in which counselling expertise may be gained by the health professional. The rest is up to the individual or the group. Good luck!

13 Extract from a counselling conversation

This annotated extract of a counsellor/client discussion is offered as an example of one way in which counselling may be conducted. It is not claimed to be typical of counselling (although many of the interventions used by the counsellor are used by many counsellors). It is offered as an illustration of some counselling interventions and as the focus of possible discussion about the hows and whys of counselling. Most of the interventions illustrated in this sample are discussed in earlier chapters.

The conversation described here is free-ranging and exploratory in nature. Conversations that took place later might be more focused. The early stages of counselling are often 'ground clearing' in nature: they allow the client to open up and begin to explore a range of issues. Often the 'real' issues don't emerge until the client has been allowed to 'wander' a little through a number of issues.

Counsellor: Hello, how can I help?[1]

Client: Well, I don't know really. I just need to talk some things through. I don't really know where to start.[2]

Counsellor: Tell me a little bit about yourself.[3]

Client: I'm 32, married with two small children. I work as a nursing assistant in a small cottage hospital. We've been married for ten years and . . . things . . . aren't working out . . .[4]

Counsellor: Things aren't working out . . .[5]

Client: Well, not properly. Me and my wife are unhappy with the way things are at the moment.

Counsellor: What's your wife's name?[6]

Client: Jane. She says she's happy enough but I don't really think we communicate very well.

Counsellor: Jane says she's happy enough . . .[7]

Client: She hasn't actually said that but I always get the impression that things are all right for her. On the other hand, we don't talk very much to each other. We sort of live parallel lives, I think.

Counsellor: What do you *need* to talk about?[8]

[1] Broad, opening question. Perhaps too broad.
[2] Client has problems answering it, so . . .
[3] Counsellor asks a more specific question. The question allows the client to begin to talk about himself.
[4] After brief biographical details, client alludes to problems.
[5] Counsellor offers straight reflection.
[6] Counsellor encourages the client to *personalize* the relationship.
[7] Counsellor offers a selective reflection and picks up on the tone of voice and emphasis offered by the client.
[8] This is a slightly confronting and challenging question. Counsellor tries to get to specifics.

Client: Almost everything! How we feel about each other and the children. Our relationship . . . sex. Everything really[9]

Counsellor: Was there a time when you did talk to each other?[10]

Client: Yes. We always used to talk . . . When we first got married, we talked about everything we did. We had no secrets from each other and we used to go out about twice and week and we couldn't stop talking. Now we can't really *start*!

Counsellor: When did you stop?[11]

Client: We just drifted into it, I suppose . . . you know how it is . . .

Counsellor: There was nothing, particular, that stopped you. . .?[12]

Client: Well, yes, there was. I . . . I had an affair a couple of years ago. I met this girl at work and we got quite serious for a while. I ended up telling Jane and she was, obviously, very upset – so was I – and we talked about it all . . . She reckoned she forgave me . . . I'm not sure she has . . .[13]

Counsellor: You're not sure she forgave you . . .[14]

Client: No. I know she hasn't. She brings it up, sometimes, when we have an argument. She sort of throws it in my face. She hated Sarah . . . I suppose I can't blame her. I suppose I would hate it if Jane had an affair . . .

Counsellor: Would you?[15]

Client: (Laughs nervously): I was just wondering about that! It sounds awful, but sometimes I wish she would have an affair. That would sort of even things up. It would make things a bit more balanced.

Counsellor: It would make you feel better?[16]

Client: I suppose so. I feel really guilty about what happened with Sarah.[17]

Counsellor.: *What did* happen?[18]

Client: Well, we talked about setting up together. At one stage, I was going to leave Jane and move in with Sarah.

Counsellor: Did you discuss that with Jane?

[9] Client's response suggests that the intervention may have been *too* direct. His response suggests that *everything* needs to be talked about.

[10] As a result, counsellor 'backs off' a little and asks a more general question about communication.

[11] Now, counsellor returns to a very specific and challenging question.

[12] Counsellor, picking up on non-verbal behaviour, persists in trying to focus the conversation.

[13] Considerable disclosure on the part of the client and first indication of what may be at the heart of some of the problems.

[14] Counsellor offers a reflection on the issue of forgiveness.

[15] A challenge from the counsellor. The client's statement is checked and seems to strike a chord.

[16] A slightly judgemental response from the counsellor.

[17] Client's response may be in direct response to counsellor's slightly judgemental tone. Counsellor notes this and moves on . . .

[18] Counsellor invites client to be specific about the relationship.

Client: No, not at all. Me and Sarah used to talk about it a lot. Sarah wasn't married or anything – she was only young . . . 18 . . . and she reckoned we could live together and that it would all work out . . .
Counsellor: So what happened[19]?
Client: She gave me an ultimatum. Either I told Jane that I was leaving her or *she* would leave . . .
Counsellor: And you chose to stay with Jane?
Client: Yes. I told Sarah that I wasn't going to leave her and the children. I *couldn't* leave . . . it would have been the end of things . . .
Counsellor: What's happening now. . . ?[20]
Client: I'm feeling upset . . . I'm a bit embarrassed . . . I think . . . .(begins to cry)
Counsellor: It's OK if you cry . . . you're allowed to have feelings . . . .[21]
Client: I just . . . bottled them up a bit, I suppose . . . I just sort of froze after we finished and I went back home . . . I just couldn't settle back down with Jane. I felt guilty . . .[22]
Counsellor: And how are you feeling now?[23]
Client: Still guilty . . . I wish I hadn't messed things up at home. It wasn't fair to Jane or the children . . .
Counsellor: Or to you?
Client: No, I suppose not. Though I chose to go out with Sarah . . . no one made me do it![24]
Counsellor: Why did you?
Client: Because I liked her. She had a sense of humour and she liked me. We got on well together and everything. It just sort of happened . . .
Counsellor: But you *chose* to go out with her?[25]
Client: Yes, I can remember that. I can remember the day when I made that decision . . .[26]
Counsellor: Can you describe it?[27]
Client: I was at work and she came on duty. We talked a bit over coffee and everything and she kept looking at me and smiling. I can remember . . . it was 3.30 . . . and I said . . . (begins to cry again) . . . I asked her if she would go out with me . . .
Counsellor: That was a tough decision?[28]

[19] Again, counsellor looks for specifics and helps client to focus the discussion.
[20] At this point, the client looks at the floor and his tone of voice and facial colour change. The counsellor notes these non-verbal changes and asks the client what is happening . . .
[21] Counsellor 'gives permission' to the client . . .
[22] Client identifies a mixture of feelings.
[23] Counsellor brings client to the 'present time'. It might be possible to return to the feelings 'in the past' later in the counselling session. At this point, though, the counsellor has made a decision to return to the present.
[24] Client accepts 'responsibility' for the relationship.
[25] Counsellor persists with the 'responsibility' issue, perhaps a little too much . . .
[26] On the other hand, it leads client to a specific remembrance.
[27] Counsellor invites client to offer a 'literal description' of the events of the time. Sometimes such invitations lead to further cathartic (emotional) release.
[28] Counsellor offers an empathy-building statement. If it is 'right', the client will agree . . .

Client: It was horrible, looking back! I should never have said it . . . I fancied her . . . I thought I loved her at the time . . .
Counsellor: Did you love her?[29]
Client: Yes! That's the problem . . . I did love her . . .
Counsellor: What's happening now. . .?[30]
Client: I feel sort of angry . . .
Counsellor: Who with?
Client: Sarah . . . (goes quiet) . . . me . . .
Counsellor: You're angry with yourself . . .[31]
Client: With both of us. We were like adolescents! She *was* adolescent, sort of . . .
Counsellor: And you were older . . .[32]
Client: I suppose I should have known better. I *was* older.
Counsellor: And because you were older, you were supposed to be in control. . . ?
Client: I suppose it doesn't work quite like that, does it? I suppose we were both responsible in some ways for what happened.
Counsellor: What was happening at home, with Jane?[33]
Client: Nothing much. We were getting on OK. The children were quite small and Jane was caught up with them. She gave up work around that time and gave all her time to them.
Counsellor: Leaving you out?[34]
Client: (grins): That's awful, isn't it? Yes, I suppose I felt left out . . . Sarah was there at the right – the *wrong* time . . . and we just . . .
Counsellor: How do you feel about Sarah now? If you met her again. . . ?[35]
Client: I wouldn't want to. It wouldn't work, now. We wouldn't have much in common any more. I've changed . . .
Counsellor: You *and* Jane have changed?
Client: Yes, I think so.
Counsellor: Does it all date back to when you were going out with Sarah?
Client: Not completely. It goes back further than that.
Counsellor: Let me just check where we've got to so far. You feel that you and Jane aren't communicating and, on the one hand, you feel that this dates back to when you met Sarah. On the other, you feel that it goes back much further. . . ?[36]

[29] Challenging and confronting question from the counsellor.
[30] Again, counsellor notes non-verbal changes and invites client to verbalize what is happening . . .
[31] Counsellor offers a mixture of reflection and empathy-building.
[32] Counsellor finishes client's sentence . . .
[33] Counsellor changes tack and asks about the 'home' situation.
[34] Counsellor seems to respond to an unspoken thought and to the client's non-verbal behaviours.
[35] Counsellor checks 'present time' feelings.
[36] The counsellor offers a summary of what has been talked about, so far. In this respect, the counsellor is *checking for understanding*.

Client: Yes, that's it, so far. I guess a lot of it has to do with things that happened way back . . . Those things are going to be more difficult to talk about . . .
Counsellor: Well, we can make a start . . .[37]

Certain key issues are demonstrated in the text.

- The counsellor 'takes the lead' from the client and 'follows' him.
- The counsellor listens not only to the words that the client uses but also to the non-verbal signals.
- The counsellor clarifies what she does not understand or follow.
- The counsellor is prepared to challenge issues raised by the client.
- The counsellor, by her approach, indicates that anything can be talked about and that feelings can be expressed.

[37] The counsellor indicates an openness to listening to 'anything' and quietly gives the client permission to talk further and deeper.

14 Conclusion

This book has covered a range of aspects of counselling skills in the health professions. This final chapter offers a summary of the main points. They are offered as a list, perhaps for discussion. Certainly there are few 'laws' of counselling and this list must necessarily be provisional and open to revision. In the end, it is my contention that the counsellor is functioning best when she 'stays out of the way' of the client and encourages the client to find their own way through. In this respect, the counsellor is a fellow-traveller, a supportive friend who nevertheless is able to keep a certain detachment and not get drawn too deeply into the client's own distress. The degree to which such detachment is possible is debatable. If the counsellor 'stands too far back' then she will be unable to empathize. If the counsellor is too close to the client, then she will be drawn into the client's life drama and be unable to provide sufficient support. Here is the list of basic issues in counselling in the health care professions.

- There is a useful distinction to be made between *counselling* and *counselling skills*. The person who works as a counsellor may do so as a full or part-time job. If asked, she may say that her job is 'a counsellor'. On the other hand, a wide range of people – both within and outside the health care professions – may find counselling skills very useful in their everyday practice. You don't have to be a counsellor to use counselling skills. Conversely, the counsellor will depend on counselling skills as part of her everyday role. It seems likely that most health professionals will use counselling skills in their work without necessarily offering full-scale counselling.
- The key issue in counselling and in the use of counselling skills is *listening*. It is the bedrock of all effective counselling and all those who work in the health care profession will benefit from constantly paying attention to the effectiveness of their listening.
- The aim of counselling should be to listen and to understand the client's point of view. It should not be to moralize or interpret, nor to offer detailed advice. While it is tempting to develop all sorts of psychological theories about why people are the way they are and why they do the things that they do, in the end it seems more appropriate, to me, to listen to the other person and to try to discover *their* theory about why and what they do. In the end, few people live their lives according to a particular psychological theory. On the other hand, we all develop a sort of personal theory about the world which guides us. The client's personal theory is the key to understanding what it is that they do in their lives.

- Counselling needs a *light touch*. If the atmosphere in a counselling session becomes too heavy and earnest, it is unlikely that much real work will be done. The counsellor who is able to keep the atmosphere relatively 'light' is, almost paradoxically, likely to enable the client to self-disclose and to express emotion far more easily.
- The outcome of counselling should be *action*. Counselling that is only about talking will not suffice. In the end, if we want our lives to be different then we must change. The action and change parts of counselling are often the most difficult, for the client and for the counsellor.
- Counselling skills can be *learned*. While most people are attracted to counselling because they are interested in other people and, presumably, already have some of the personal qualities necessary for being effective, most can also benefit from learning some of the simple skills described in this book. Learning to listen, to ask open questions, to reflect and to offer empathy may seem too simple. In the end, though, they are probably more effective than any amount of advice giving and judgement.
- A distinction can be made between *information giving* and *advice giving*. Information giving involves offering clear information about a certain topic. Thus, to the person who is worried about HIV/AIDS, information about safe sex can be useful. Advice giving, on the other hand, involves the counsellor in making some sort of moral judgement about what is right for the client and passing that on to him. Most advice is likely to follow the 'if I were you . . .' pattern. Arguably, it is far less useful, in counselling, than is information giving. It is important to be clear on the two issues.
- Counselling can be *tiring*. To listen to other people's problems and not to judge can be a draining job. Just being an effective listener takes up a considerable amount of energy. Those who work as counsellors or who regularly use counselling skills should also take care of themselves. If they do regular counselling, they should consider having a *supervisor* who will listen to and support them. Others should make sure that there are parts of their jobs which are entirely different from counselling. Full-time commitment to other people can lead to *burnout* and it is vital that all health care professionals also care for themselves.
- Counselling is learned by *doing*. You cannot learn counselling from a book. Workshops and courses which encourage *experiential learning* – learning through trying things out and then through reflection – are particularly useful. It is also important to continuously monitor your own work as a counsellor. Personal styles of counselling modify and change as the counsellor develops. On the other hand, it is also possible to slip into some bad habits in counselling. For that reason, it is useful every so often to take some sort of refresher course in counselling. It is also important to supplement practical 'hands-on' experience with plenty of reading about

the topic. While counselling cannot be learned from a book, books obviously have their part to play in informing practice.

- There remains a nagging doubt and a question: does counselling *work*? While all the anecdotal evidence suggests that it does, for some people, there remains a need for further *outcome studies* to be conducted in the field of counselling. We must remain open minded and humble about the degree to which we know that counselling makes a difference. While it seems obvious to most of us that talking about problems helps, there is to date precious little hard evidence that counselling is the prime means of helping people to come to terms with their psychological, emotional and social problems.
- Linked to the previous point is the danger that we might tend to see *emotional expression* as somehow better than *rationality*. This, in a way, has been a dogma of the past two decades. Ferguson (1998), in a widesweeping review of the past 20 years makes these comments.

> *. . . the change taking place was that the media, keeping pace with the death of argument and alleged 'end of history', had almost wholly stopped asking people 'What do you think?' and began demanding, instead, 'How do you feel?'. This was a disaster in almost every way.*
>
> *First, it established an orthodoxy of grieving that soon became the centralist norm, and later brought with it a dangerous corollary, what you might call the inviolacy of grief.*
>
> *There grew a tacit understanding that, after a tragedy or disaster, every victim was automatically brave, every perpetrator automatically evil, every reaction one of devastation: and further analysis, further thought, trying to expose a complex issue to a little rigour, would bring automatic opprobrium.*

There might just be an argument that we gain in life by suffering just as much as we do from expressing our feelings; that talking about things does not necessarily and automatically change them. There might also be an argument, sometimes, for coolly and rationally looking at our situation and making life decisions based on such rationality rather than on immediate, emotional reactions, as has in some cases become the norm. This is not at all to deny the place and value of counselling and interpersonal communication but to serve as an astringent to the view that expression of feelings and of almost *everything* is necessarily and always a good thing. We need, perhaps, to proceed with caution.

APPENDIX

Permission to reproduce the four documents on the following pages has been granted by the British Association for Counselling. The Association asks readers to note that the BAC updates these Codes on a regular basis and readers must check with BAC in order to ascertain that the particular Code printed is the latest available. Copies can be obtained from:

British Association for Counselling
1 Regent Place
Rugby
Warwickshire
CV21 2PJ

Office: 01788 550899
Information Line: 01788 578328
e-mail: bac@bac.co.uk

For Counsellors

1. *Status of this Code*

In response to the experience of members of BAC, this code is a revision of the (1992) 1993 code, amended by the Management Committee (May 1996).

2. *Introduction*

2.1 The purpose of this code is to establish and maintain standards for counsellors who are members of BAC, and to inform and protect people who seek or use their services.

2.2 All members of this Association are required to abide by the current codes appropriate to them. Implicit in these codes is a common frame of reference within which members manage their responsibilities to clients, colleagues, members of BAC and the wider community. No code can resolve all issues relating to ethics and practice. In this code we aim to provide a framework for addressing ethical issues and encouraging best possible levels of practice. Members must determine which parts apply to particular settings, taking account of any conflicting responsibilities.

2.3 The Association has a Complaints Procedure which can lead to the expulsion of members for breaches of its Codes of Ethics and Practice.

3. *The Nature of Counselling*

3.1 The overall aim of counselling is to provide an opportunity for the client to work towards living in a way he or she experiences as more satisfying and resourceful. The term 'counselling' includes work with individuals, pairs or groups of people often, but not always, referred to as 'clients'. The objectives of particular counselling relationships will vary according to the client's needs. Counselling may be concerned with developmental issues, addressing and resolving specific problems, making decisions, coping with crisis, developing personal insight and knowledge, working through feelings of inner conflict or improving relationships with others. The counsellor's role is to facilitate the client's work in ways which respect the client's values, personal resources and capacity for choice within his or her cultural context.

3.2 Counselling involves a deliberately undertaken contract with clearly agreed boundaries and commitment to privacy and confidentiality. It requires explicit and informed agreement. The use of counselling skills in other contexts, paid or voluntary, is subject to the Code of Ethics and Practice for Counselling Skills.

3.3 There is no generally accepted distinction between counselling and psychotherapy. There are well founded traditions which use the terms interchangeably and others which distinguish between them. Regardless of the theoretical approaches preferred by individual counsellors, there are ethical issues which are common to all counselling situations.

continued . . .

BRITISH ASSOCIATION
for
COUNSELLING
1 Regent Place
Rugby CV21 2PJ
Office: 01788 550899
Fax: 01788 562189
Minicom: 01788 572838
e-mail: bac@bac.co.uk

Code of Ethics & Practice

1 January 1998

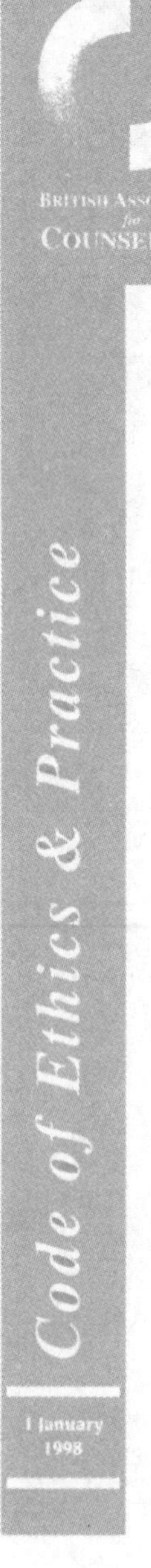

4. Equal Opportunities Policy Statement

All BAC members abide by its Equal Opportunities Policy statement. The full statement can be found at the end of this Code.

5. The Structure of this Code

This code has been divided into two parts. The Code of Ethics outlines the fundamental values of counselling and a number of general principles arising from these. The Code of Practice applies these principles to the counselling situation.

A. CODE OF ETHICS

Values
Counsellors' basic values are integrity, impartiality and respect.

A.1 Responsibility
All reasonable steps should be taken to ensure the client's safety during counselling sessions. Counselling is a non-exploitative activity. Counsellors must take the same degree of care to work ethically whatever the setting or the financial basis of the counselling contract.

A.2 Anti-discriminatory Practice
Counsellors must consider and address their own prejudices and stereotyping and ensure that an anti-discriminatory approach is integral to their counselling practice.

A.3 Confidentiality
Counsellors offer the highest possible levels of confidentiality in order to respect the client's privacy and create the trust necessary for counselling.

A.4 Contracts
The terms and conditions on which counselling is offered shall be made clear to clients before counselling begins. Subsequent revision of these terms should be agreed in advance of any changes.

A.5 Boundaries
Counsellors must establish and maintain appropriate boundaries around the counselling relationship. Counsellors must take into account the effects of any overlapping or pre-existing relationships.

A.6 Competence
Counsellors shall take all reasonable steps to monitor and develop their own competence and to work within the limits of that competence. Counsellors must have appropriate, regular and ongoing counselling supervision.

B. CODE OF PRACTICE

Introduction
This code applies these values and ethical principles outlined above to more specific situations which may arise in the practice of counselling. The sections and clauses are arranged in the order of the ethics section and under the same headings. No clause or section should be read in isolation from the rest of the Code.

B.1 Issues of Responsibility

B.1.1 The counsellor-client relationship is the foremost ethical concern. However, counselling does not exist in social isolation. Counsellors may need to consider other sources of ethical responsibility. The headings in this section are intended to draw attention to some of these.

B.1.2 Counsellors take responsibility for clinical/therapeutic decisions in their work with clients.

B.1.3 Responsibility to the Client

continued. . .

Client Safety

B.1.3.1 Counsellors must take all reasonable steps to ensure that the client suffers neither physical nor psychological harm during counselling sessions.

B.1.3.2 Counsellors must not exploit their clients financially, sexually, emotionally, or in any other way. Suggesting or engaging in sexual activity with a client is unethical.

B.1.3.3 Counsellors must provide privacy for counselling sessions. The sessions should not be overheard, recorded or observed by anyone other than the counsellor without informed consent from the client. Normally any recording would be discussed as part of the contract. Care must be taken that sessions are not interrupted.

Client Self-determination

B.1.3.4 In counselling the balance of power is unequal and counsellors must take care not to abuse their power.

B.1.3.5 Counsellors do not normally act on behalf of their clients. If they do, it will be only at the express request of the client, or else in exceptional circumstances..

B.1.3.6 Counsellors do not normally give advice.

B1.3.7 Counsellors have a responsibility to establish with clients, at the outset of counselling, the existence of any other therapeutic or helping relationships in which the client is involved and to consider whether counselling is appropriate. Counsellors should gain the client's permission before conferring in any way with other professional workers.

Breaks and Endings

B.1.3.8 Counsellors work with clients to reach a recognised ending when clients have received the help they sought or when it is apparent that counselling is no longer helping or when clients wish to end.

B.1.3.9 External circumstances may lead to endings for other reasons which are not therapeutic. Counsellors must make arrangements for care to be taken of the immediate needs of clients in the event of any sudden and unforeseen endings by the counsellor or breaks to the counselling relationship.

B.1.3.10 Counsellors should take care to prepare their clients appropriately for any planned breaks from counselling. They should take any necessary steps to ensure the well-being of their clients during such breaks.

B.1.4 Responsibility to other Counsellors

B.1.4.1 Counsellors must not conduct themselves in their counselling-related activities in ways which undermine public confidence either in their role as a counsellor or in the work of other counsellors.

B.1.4.2 A counsellor who suspects misconduct by another counsellor, which cannot be resolved or remedied after discussion with the counsellor concerned, should implement the Complaints Procedure, doing so without breaches of confidentiality other than those necessary for investigating the complaint.

B.1.5 Responsibility to Colleagues and Others

B.1.5.1 Counsellors are accountable for their services to colleagues, employers and funding bodies as appropriate. At the same time they must respect the privacy, needs and autonomy of the client as well as the contract of confidentiality agreed with the client.

B.1.5.2 No-one should be led to believe that a service is being offered by the counsellor which is not in fact being offered as this may deprive the client of the offer of such a service from elsewhere.

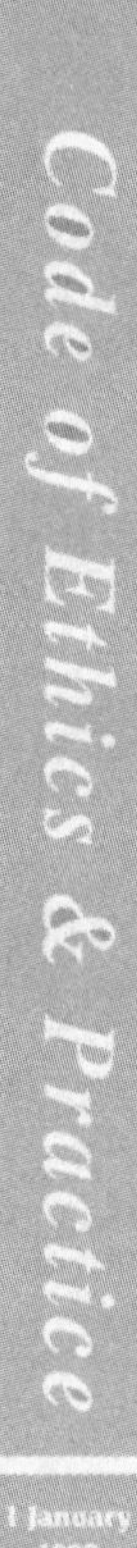

continued . . .

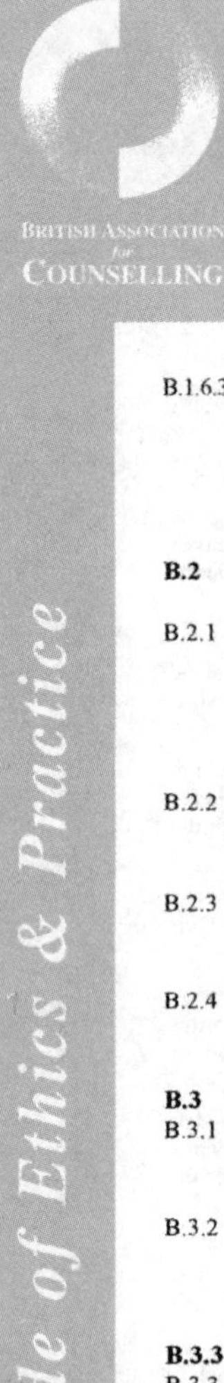

B.1.5.3 Counsellors must play a demonstrable part in exploring and resolving conflicts of interest between themselves and their employers or agencies, especially where this affects the ethical delivery of counselling to clients.

B.1.6 Responsibility to the Wider Community

Law

B.1.6.1 Counsellors must take all reasonable steps to be aware of current law as it applies to their counselling practice. (See BAC Information Guide 1 'Counselling, Confidentiality and the Law').

Research

B.1.6.2 Counsellors must conduct any research in accordance with BAC guidelines (see BAC Information Guide 4 'Ethical Guidelines for Monitoring, Evaluation and Research in Counselling').

Resolving Conflicts between Ethical Priorities

B.1.6.3 Counsellors may find themselves caught between conflicting ethical principles, which could involve issues of public interest. In these circumstances, they are urged to consider the particular situation in which they find themselves and to discuss the situation with their counselling supervisor and/or other experienced counsellors. Even after conscientious consideration of the salient issues, some ethical dilemmas cannot be resolved easily or wholly satisfactorily.

B.2 Anti-discriminatory Practice

Client Respect

B.2.1 Counsellors work with clients in ways that affirm both the common humanity and the uniqueness of each individual.

They must be sensitive to the cultural context and world view of the client, for instance whether the individual, family or the community is taken as central.

Client Autonomy

B.2.2 Counsellors are responsible for working in ways which respect and promote the client's ability to make decisions in the light of his/her own beliefs, values and context.

Counsellor Awareness

B.2.3 Counsellors are responsible for ensuring that any problems with mutual comprehension due to language, cultural differences or for any other reason are addressed at an early stage. The use of an interpreter needs to be carefully considered at the outset of counselling.

B.2.4 Counsellors have a responsibility to consider and address their own prejudices and stereotyping attitudes and behaviour and particularly to consider ways in which these may be affecting the counselling relationship and influencing their responses.

B.3 Confidentiality

B.3.1 Confidentiality is a means of providing the client with safety and privacy and thus protects client autonomy. For this reason any limitation on the degree of confidentiality is likely to diminish the effectiveness of counselling.

B.3.2 The counselling contract will include an agreement about the level and limits of confidentiality offered. This agreement can be reviewed and changed by negotiation between counsellor and client. Agreements about confidentiality continue after the client's death unless there are overriding legal or ethical considerations.

B.3.3 Settings

B.3.3.1 Counsellors must ensure that they have taken all reasonable steps to inform the client of any limitations to confidentiality that arise within the setting of the counselling work e.g updating doctors in primary care, team case discussion in agencies. These are made explicit through clear contracting.

continued . . .

B.3.3.2 Many settings place additional specific limitations on confidentiality. Counsellors considering working in these settings must think about the impact of such limitations on their practice and decide whether or not to work in such settings.

B.3.4 Exceptional Circumstances

B.3.4.1 Exceptional circumstances may arise which give the counsellor good grounds for believing that serious harm may occur to the client or to other people. In such circumstances the client's consent to a change in the agreement about confidentiality should be sought whenever possible unless there are also good grounds for believing the client is no longer willing or able to take responsibility for his/her actions. Normally, the decision to break confidentiality should be discussed with the client and should be made only after consultation with the counselling supervisor or if he/she is not available, an experienced counsellor.

B.3.4.2 Any disclosure of confidential information should be restricted to relevant information, conveyed only to appropriate people and for appropriate reasons likely to alleviate the exceptional circumstances. The ethical considerations include achieving a balance between acting in the best interests of the client and the counsellor's responsibilities to the wider community.

B.3.4.3 Counsellors hold different views about the grounds for breaking confidentiality, such as potential self-harm, suicide, and harm to others. Counsellors must consider their own views, as they will affect their practice and communicate them to clients and significant others e.g supervisor, agency.

B.3.5 Management of Confidentiality

B.3.5.1 Counsellors should ensure that records of the client's identity are kept separately from any case notes.

B.3.5.2 Arrangements must be made for the safe disposal of client records, especially in the event of the counsellor's incapacity or death.

B.3.5.3 Care must be taken to ensure that personally identifiable information is not transmitted through overlapping networks of confidential relationships.

B.3.5.4 When case material is used for case studies, reports or publications the client's informed consent must be obtained wherever possible and their identity must be effectively disguised.

B.3.5.5 Any discussion about their counselling work between the counsellor and others should be purposeful and not trivialising.

B.3.5.6 Counsellors must pay particular attention to protecting the identity of clients. This includes discussion of cases in counselling supervision.

B.4 Contracts

B.4.1 Advertising & Public Statements

B.4.1.1 Membership of BAC is not a qualification and it must not be used as if it were. In press advertisements and telephone directories, on business cards, letterheads, brass plates and plaques etc counsellors should limit the information to name, relevant qualifications, address, telephone number, hours available, a listing of the services offered and fees charged. They should not mention membership of BAC.

B.4.1.2 In oral statements, letters and pre-counselling leaflets to the public and potential clients, BAC membership may not be mentioned without a statement that it means that the individual, and where appropriate the organisation, abides by the Codes of Ethics and Practice and is subject to the Complaints Procedure of the British Association for Counselling. Copies of these Codes and the Complaints Procedure are available from BAC.

British Association for Counselling

Code of Ethics & Practice

1 January 1998

continued . . .

BRITISH ASSOCIATION for COUNSELLING

Code of Ethics & Practice

1 January 1998

B.4.1.3 Counsellors who are accredited and/or registered are encouraged to mention this.

B.4.1.4 All advertising and public statements should be accurate in every particular.

B.4.1.5 Counsellors should not display an affiliation with an organisation in a manner which falsely implies sponsorship or validation by that organisation

B.4.2 Pre-counselling information

B.4.2.1 Any publicity material and all written and oral information should reflect accurately the nature of the service on offer, and the relevant counselling training, qualifications and experience of the counsellor.

B.4.2.2 Counsellors should take all reasonable steps to honour undertakings made in their pre-counselling information

B.4.3 Contracting with Clients

B.4.3.1 Counsellors are responsible for reaching agreement with their clients about the terms on which counselling is being offered, including availability, the degree of confidentiality offered, arrangements for the payment of any fees, cancelled appointments and other significant matters. The communication of essential terms and any negotiations should be concluded by having reached a clear agreement before the client incurs any commitment or liability of any kind.

B.4.3.2 The counsellor has a responsibility to ensure that the client is given a free choice whether or not to participate in counselling. Reasonable steps should be taken in the course of the counselling relationship to ensure that the client is given an opportunity to review the counselling.

B.4.3.3 Counsellors must avoid conflicts of interest wherever possible. Any conflicts of interest that do occur must be discussed in counselling supervision and where appropriate with the client.

B.4.3.4 Records of appointments should be kept and clients should be made aware of this. If records of counselling sessions are kept, clients should also be made aware of this. At the client's request information should be given about access to these records, their availability to other people, and the degree of security with which they are kept.

B.4.3.5 Counsellors must be aware that computer-based records are subject to statutory regulations. It is the counsellor's responsibility to be aware of any changes the government may introduce in the regulations concerning the client's right of access to his/her records

B.4.3.6 Counsellors are responsible for addressing any client dissatisfaction with the counselling.

B.5 Boundaries

With Clients

B.5.1 Counsellors are responsible for setting and monitoring boundaries throughout the counselling sessions and will make explicit to clients that counselling is a formal and contracted relationship and nothing else.

B.5.2 The counselling relationship must not be concurrent with a supervisory or training relationship.

With Former Clients

B.5.3 Counsellors remain accountable for relationships with former clients and must exercise caution over entering into friendships, business relationships, sexual relationships, training, supervising and other relationships. Any changes in relationship must be discussed in counselling supervision. The decision about any change(s) in relationship with former clients should take into account whether the issues and power dynamics present during the counselling relationship have been resolved.

continued . . .

B.5.4 Counsellors who belong to organisations which prohibit sexual activity with all former clients are bound by that commitment.

B.6 Competence

B.6.1 Counsellor Competence

B.6.1.1 Counsellors must have achieved a level of competence before commencing counselling and must maintain continuing professional development as well as regular and ongoing supervision.

B.6.1.2 Counsellors must actively monitor their own competence through counselling supervision and be willing to consider any views expressed by their clients and by other counsellors.

B.6.1.3 Counsellors will monitor their functioning and will not counsel when their functioning is impaired by alcohol or drugs. In situations of personal or emotional difficulty, or illness, counsellors will monitor the point at which they are no longer competent to practise and take action accordingly.

B.6.1.4 Competence includes being able to recognise when it is appropriate to refer a client elsewhere.

B.6.1.5 Counsellors are responsible for ensuring that their relationships with clients are not unduly influenced by their own emotional needs.

B.6.1.6 Counsellors must consider the need for professional indemnity insurance and when appropriate take out and maintain adequate cover.

B.6.1.7 When uncertain as to whether a particular situation or course of action may be in violation of the Code of Ethics and Practice, counsellors must consult with their counselling supervisor and/or other experienced practitioners.

B.6.2 Counsellor Safety

B.6.2.1 Counsellors should take all reasonable steps to ensure their own physical safety.

B.6.3 Counselling Supervision

B.6.3.1 Counselling supervision refers to a formal arrangement which enables counsellors to discuss their counselling regularly with one or more people who are normally experienced as counselling practitioners and have an understanding of counselling supervision. Its purpose is to ensure the efficacy of the counsellor-client relationship. It is a confidential relationship.

B.6.3.2 The counselling supervisor role should wherever possible be independent of the line manager role. However, where the counselling supervisor is also the line manager, the counsellor must have additional regular access to independent counselling supervision.

B.6.3.3 Counselling supervision must be regular, consistent and appropriate to the counselling. The volume should reflect the volume of counselling work undertaken and the experience of the counsellor.

B.6.4 Awareness of Other Codes

Counsellors must take account of the following Codes and Procedures adopted by the Annual General Meetings of the British Association for Counselling:

Code of Ethics & Practice for Counselling Skills (1988) *applies to members who would not regard themselves as counsellors, but who use counselling skills to support other roles.*

Code of Ethics & Practice for Supervisors of Counsellors (1996) *applies to members offering supervision to counsellors and also helps counsellors seeking supervision.*

Code of Ethics & Practice for Trainers (1997) *applies to members offering training to counsellors and also helps members of the public seeking counselling training.*

Complaints Procedure (1997) *applies to members of BAC in the event of complaints about breaches of the Codes of Ethics & Practice.*

continued . . .

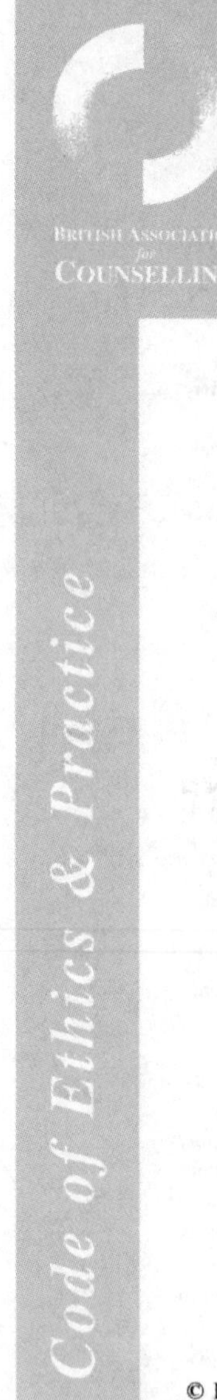

Copies and other guidelines and information sheets relevant to maintaining ethical standards of practice can be obtained from the BAC office, 1 Regent Place, Rugby CV21 2PJ.

Equal Opportunities Policy Statement

The 'British Association for Counselling' (BAC) is committed to promoting Equality of Opportunity of access and participation for all its members in all of its structures and their workings. BAC has due regard for those groups of people with identifiable characteristics which can lead to visible and invisible barriers thus inhibiting their joining and full participation in BAC. Barriers can include age, colour, creed, culture, disability, education, 'ethnicity', gender, information, knowledge, mobility, money, nationality, race, religion, sexual orientation, social class and status.

The work of BAC aims to reflect this commitment in all area including services to members, employer responsibilities, the recruitment of and working with volunteers, setting, assessing, monitoring and evaluating standards and the implementation of the complaints procedures. This is particularly important as BAC is the 'Voice of Counselling' in the wider world.

BAC will promote and encourage commitment to Equality of Opportunity by its members.

Effective from 1 January 1998

8

For Trainers

British Association for Counselling
1 Regent Place
Rugby CV21 2PJ
Office: 01788 550899
Fax: 01788 562189

Code of Ethics & Practice

January 1997

1. Status of this Code

1.1 In response to the experience of members of BAC, this Code is a revision of the 1996 Code.

Structure of this Code

This code is in four sections:

A. A Code of Ethics for all Trainers.

B. A general Code of Practice for all Trainers.

C. Additional clause for Trainers in Counselling.

D. Additional clauses for Trainers in Counselling Skills

2. Introduction

2.1 The purpose of this Code of Ethics and Practice is to establish and maintain standards for trainers who are members of BAC and to inform and protect members of the public seeking training in counselling, counselling skills or counselling-related areas, whatever the level or length of the training programme. Training in counselling-related areas includes training in counselling supervision, group work, interpersonal skills and other topics involving counselling theory and practice.

Sections A and B apply to all trainers. Section C contains an additional clause for trainers in counselling. Section D contains additional clauses for trainers in counselling skills.

2.2 The document must be seen in relation to all other BAC Codes of Ethics and Practice and BAC Course Recognition Procedures.

2.3 There is an important relationship between the agency employing the trainer and the trainee undertaking the training. This Code reinforces the principle that agencies which are organisational members of BAC abide by all BAC codes.

2.4 Ethical standards comprise such values as integrity, impartiality and respect. Anti-discriminatory practice reflects the basic values of counselling and training. Members of BAC, in assenting to this Code, accept their appropriate responsibilities as trainers, to trainees, trainees' clients, employing agencies, colleagues, this Association and to the wider community.

continued . . .

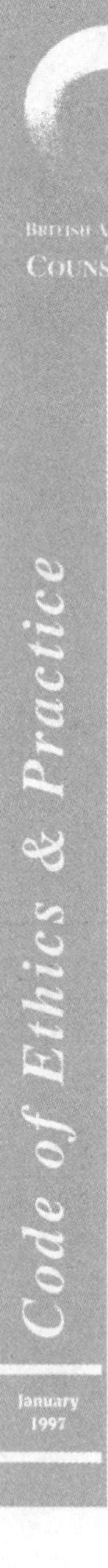

2.5 In the context of this Code, trainers are those who train people in counselling, in counselling skills or in counselling-related areas. They should be experienced and competent practitioners. Trainers have a responsibility to draw the attention of trainees to all BAC Codes of Ethics and Practice.

2.6 Trainers must be aware that there are differences between training in counselling, training in counselling skills and training in counselling-related areas. Trainees must be made aware of this and trainers should endeavour to ensure that their intending trainees join an appropriate training programme.

2.7 There should be consistency between the theoretical orientation of the programme and the training methods and, where they are used, methods of assessment and evaluation (e.g. client-centred courses would normally be trainee-centred).

2.8 Training is at its most effective when there are two or more trainers. Trainers and their employing agencies have a responsibility to ensure this wherever possible.

2.9 The size of the group must be congruent with the training objectives and the model of working. Decisions about staff:student ratios must take account of the learning objectives and methods of assessment and of the importance of being able to give individual attention and recognition to each course member. Where direct feedback between trainer and trainee is an important part of the course a maximum staff to student ratio of 1:12 is recommended best practice.

A. *Code of Ethics for All Trainers*

A.1 Values

Training is a non-exploitative activity. Its basic values are integrity, impartiality and respect. Trainers must take the same degree of care to work ethically whether the training is paid or unpaid.

A.2 Anti-discrimination

Trainers must consider and address their own prejudices and stereotyping. They must also address the prejudices and stereotyping of their trainees. They must ensure that an anti-discriminatory approach is integral to all the training they provide.

A.3 Safety

All reasonable steps shall be taken by trainers to ensure the safety of trainees and clients during training.

A.4 Competence

Trainers must take all reasonable steps to monitor and develop their competence as trainers and work within the limits of that competence.

A.5 Confidentiality

Trainers must clarify the limits of confidentiality within the training process at the beginning of the training programme.

continued . . .

A.6 Contracts

The terms and conditions on which the training is offered must be made clear to trainees before the start of the training programme. Subsequent revision of these terms must be agreed in advance of any changes.

A.7 Boundaries

Trainers must maintain and establish appropriate boundaries between themselves and their trainees so that working relationships are not confused with friendship or other relationships.

B. General Code of Practice for All Trainers

B.1 Responsibility

B.1.1 Trainers deliberately undertake the task of delivering training in counselling, counselling skills and counselling-related areas.

B.1.2 Trainers are responsible for observing the principles embodied in this Code of Ethics and Practice and all current BAC Codes and for introducing trainees to the BAC Codes of Ethics and Practice in the early stages of the training programme.

B.1.3 Trainers must recognise the value and dignity of trainees, with due regard to issues of origin, status, gender, age, beliefs, sexual preference or disability. Trainers have a responsibility to be aware of, and address their own issues of prejudice and stereotyping, and to give particular consideration to ways in which this may impact on the training.

B.1.4 Trainers have a responsibility to encourage and facilitate the self-development and self-awareness of trainees, so that trainees learn to integrate practice and personal insights.

B.1.5 Trainers are responsible for making explicit to trainees the boundaries between training, counselling supervision, consultancy, counselling and the use of counselling skills.

B.1.6 Trainers are responsible for modelling appropriate boundaries.

1.6.1 The roles of trainee and client must be kept separate during the training; where painful personal issues are revealed, trainers are responsible for suggesting and encouraging further in-depth work with a counsellor outside the training context.

1.6.2 The providers of counselling for trainees during the programme must be independent of the training context and any assessment procedures.

1.6.3 Trainers should take all reasonable steps to ensure that any personal and social contacts between them and their trainees do not adversely influence the effectiveness of the training.

B.1.7 Trainers must not accept current clients as trainees. Former trainees must not become clients, nor former clients become trainees, until a period of time has elapsed for reflection and after consultation with a counselling supervisor.

B.1.8 Trainers are responsible for ensuring that their emotional needs are met outside the training work and are not dependent on their relationships with trainees.

B.1.9 Trainers must not exploit their trainees financially, sexually, emotionally, or in any other way. Engaging in sexual activity with trainees is unethical.

continued . . .

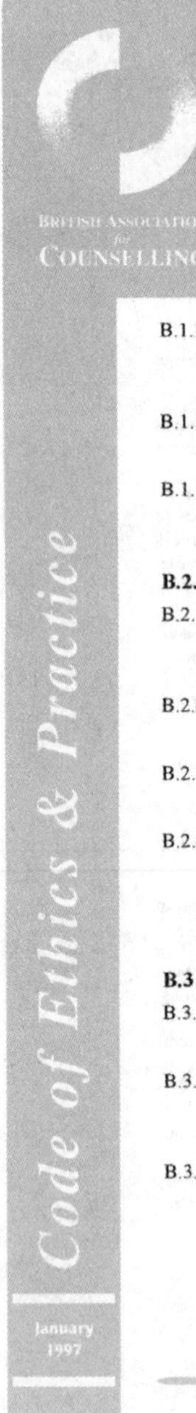

B.1.10 Trainers must ensure that consideration is given to the appropriateness of the settings in which trainees propose to, or are expected to, work on completion of the training programme.

B.1.11 Trainers are expected, when appropriate, to prepare trainees to practice effectively within their work setting.

B.1.12 Trainers have a responsibility to ensure that appropriate counselling supervision arrangements are in place for trainees where working with clients is part of the course.

B.1.13 Visiting or occasional trainers on programmes must ensure that they take responsibility for any former or current pre-existing professional or personal relationship with any member of the training group.

B.1.14 Trainers must acknowledge the individual life experience and identity of trainees. Challenges to the views, attitudes and outlooks of trainees must be respectful, related to the stated objectives of the course, and model good practice.

B.1.15 Trainers are responsible for discussing with trainees any needs for personal counselling and the contribution it might make to the trainees' work both during and after the programme.

B.1.16 Trainers must at all times conduct themselves in their training activities in ways which will not undermine public confidence in their role as trainers, in the work of other trainers or in the role of BAC.

B.2. Competence

B.2.1 It is strongly recommended that trainers should have completed at least one year's post-training experience as practitioners in an appropriate field of work. They should commit themselves to continuing professional development as trainers.

B.2.2 Trainers must monitor their training work and be able and willing to account to trainees and colleagues for what they do and why.

B.2.3 Trainers must monitor and evaluate the limits of their competence as trainers by means of regular supervision or consultancy.

B.2.4 Trainers have a responsibility to themselves and to their trainees to maintain their own effectiveness, resilience and ability to work with trainees. They are expected to monitor their own personal functioning and to seek help and/or agree to withdraw from training, whether temporarily or permanently, when their personal resources are so depleted as to require this.

B.3 Confidentiality

B.3.1 Trainers are responsible for establishing a contract for confidential working which makes explicit the responsibilities of both trainer and trainees.

B.3.2 Trainers must inform trainees at the beginning of the training programme of all reasonably foreseeable circumstances under which confidentiality may be breached during the training programme.

B.3.3 Trainers must not reveal confidential information concerning trainees, or former trainees, without the permission of the trainee, except:

a. in discussion with those on whom trainers rely for professional support and supervision. (These discussions will usually be anonymous and the supervisor is bound by confidentiality);

continued ... .

b. in order to prevent serious harm to another or to the trainee

c. when legally required to break confidentiality;

d. during selection, assessment, complaints and disciplinary procedures in order to prevent or investigate breaches of ethical standards by trainees;

If consent to the disclosure of confidential information has been withheld, trainees should normally be informed in advance that a trainer intends to disclose confidential information.

B.3.4 Detailed information about specific trainees, or former trainees, may be used for publication or in meetings only with the trainees' permission and with anonymity preserved. Where trainers need to use examples from previous work to illustrate a point to trainees, this must be done respectfully, briefly and anonymously.

B.3.5 If discussion by trainers of their trainees, or former trainees, with professional colleagues becomes necessary, it must be purposeful, not trivialising, and relevant to the training.

B.3.6 If trainers suspect misconduct by another trainer which cannot be resolved or remedied after discussion with the trainer concerned, they should implement any internal complaints procedures that may be available or the BAC Complaints Procedure. Any required breaches of confidentiality should be limited to those necessary for the investigation of the complaint.

B.4 Management of the Training Work

B.4.1 Trainers must make basic information available to potential trainees, in writing or by other appropriate means of communication, before the start of the programme. This should include:

a. the fees to be charged and any other expenses which may be incurred;

b. the dates and time commitments;

c. information on selection procedures, entry requirements and the process by which decisions are made;

d. basic information about the content of the programme, its philosophical and theoretical approach and the training methods to be used;

e. the relevant qualifications of the trainers;

f. any requirements for counselling supervision or personal counselling which trainees will be expected to comply with while training;

g. guidelines for work experience or placements to be undertaken as part of the training.

h. evaluation and assessment methods to be used during the programme and the implications of these;

i. if the programme carries a qualification, arrangements for appeals should a dispute arise.

B.4.2 Trainers must check whether training is being undertaken voluntarily or compulsorily and, if necessary, draw employers' attention to the fact that a voluntary commitment is the more appropriate.

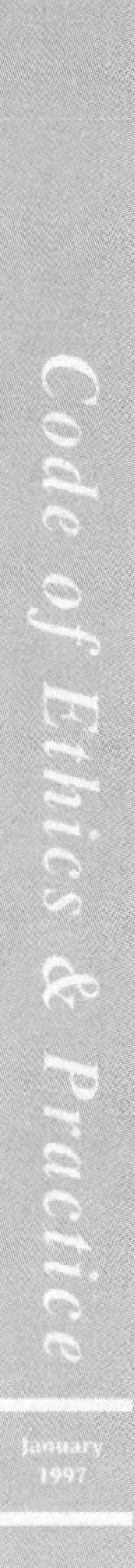

continued . . .

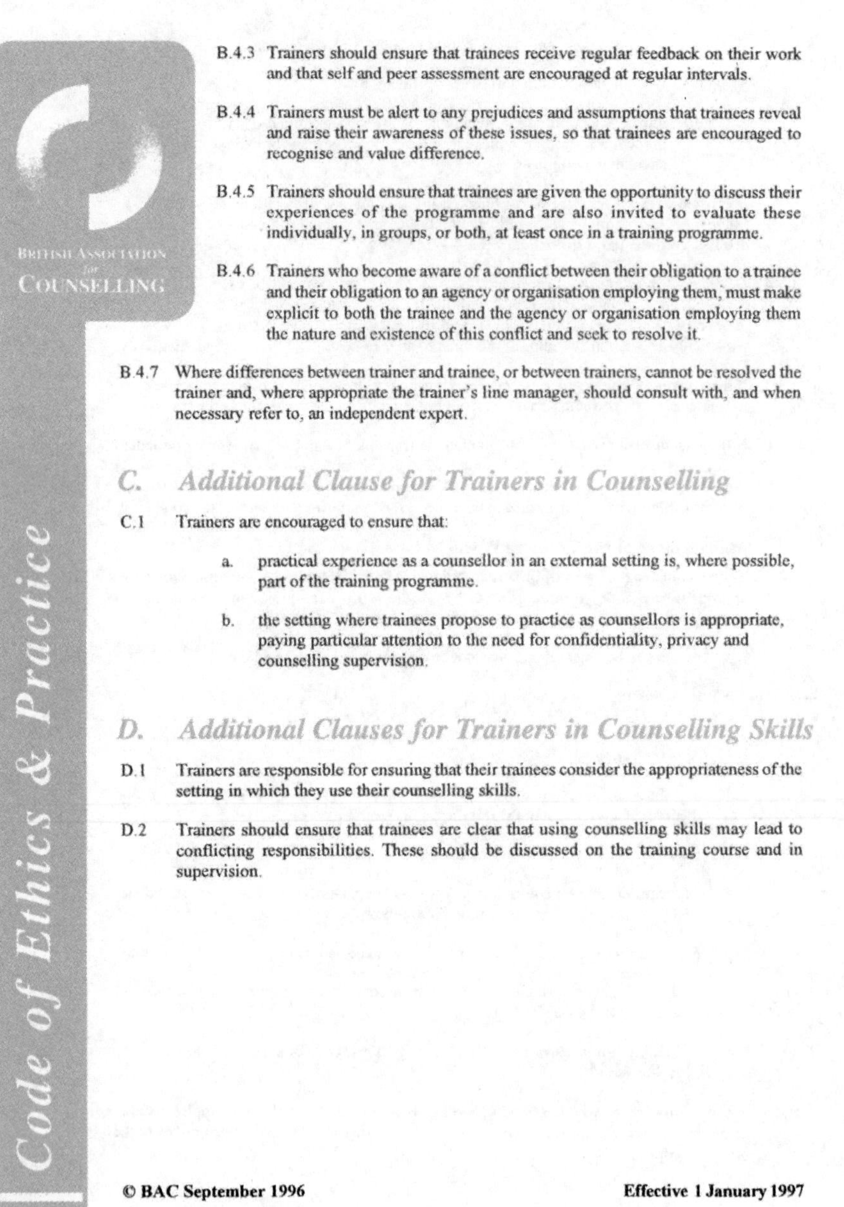

B.4.3 Trainers should ensure that trainees receive regular feedback on their work and that self and peer assessment are encouraged at regular intervals.

B.4.4 Trainers must be alert to any prejudices and assumptions that trainees reveal and raise their awareness of these issues, so that trainees are encouraged to recognise and value difference.

B.4.5 Trainers should ensure that trainees are given the opportunity to discuss their experiences of the programme and are also invited to evaluate these individually, in groups, or both, at least once in a training programme.

B.4.6 Trainers who become aware of a conflict between their obligation to a trainee and their obligation to an agency or organisation employing them, must make explicit to both the trainee and the agency or organisation employing them the nature and existence of this conflict and seek to resolve it.

B.4.7 Where differences between trainer and trainee, or between trainers, cannot be resolved the trainer and, where appropriate the trainer's line manager, should consult with, and when necessary refer to, an independent expert.

C. *Additional Clause for Trainers in Counselling*

C.1 Trainers are encouraged to ensure that:

a. practical experience as a counsellor in an external setting is, where possible, part of the training programme.

b. the setting where trainees propose to practice as counsellors is appropriate, paying particular attention to the need for confidentiality, privacy and counselling supervision.

D. *Additional Clauses for Trainers in Counselling Skills*

D.1 Trainers are responsible for ensuring that their trainees consider the appropriateness of the setting in which they use their counselling skills.

D.2 Trainers should ensure that trainees are clear that using counselling skills may lead to conflicting responsibilities. These should be discussed on the training course and in supervision.

 Effective 1 January 1997

6

Guidelines for those using Counselling Skills in their Work

Status of this Code

In response to members of BAC, this Code is a revision of the 1989 Code of Ethics and Practice for Counselling Skills. All members of this Association are required to abide by the existing Codes appropriate to their work until such time as a new Code is adopted by the membership.

British Association
Counselling

A. *Introduction*

The purpose of this Code is to outline the ethical principles involved in the use of Counselling Skills.

The attached practice guidelines which relate to this Code (Section D) are primarily intended for those who are trained in the use of Counselling Skills within another role. For those working within an explicitly contracted counselling relationship, the Code of Ethics and Practice for Counsellors applies.

The user of Counselling Skills will hereafter be known as 'the practitioner' and the recipient of Counselling Skills will be known as 'the client'.

Counselling Skills Users, their organisations, their managers and their clients should have access to this Code.

All BAC members abide by its Equal Opportunities Policy Statement. The full statement can be found at the end of this Code.

B. *Counselling Skills*

For the purpose of this Code and the Practice Guidelines:

The **practitioner** respects the client's values, experience, thoughts, feelings and their capacity for self-determination. The practitioner aims to serve the best interests of the **client**.

Counselling Skills are being used:

- **when** there is intentional use of specific interpersonal skills which reflect the values of counselling,
- **and** when the practitioner's primary role (e.g nurse, tutor, line manager, social worker, personnel officer, helper) is enhanced without being changed;
- **and** when the client perceives the practitioner as acting within their primary professional or/caring role which is **not** that of being a counsellor.

C. *Code of Ethics*

C.1 Values

The practitioner's values are those of integrity, impartiality and respect for the client. The practitioner works in a non-exploitative way.

C.2 Anti-discriminatory Practice

Practitioners must consider and address their own prejudices and how they stereotype others. They must ensure that anti-discriminatory practice is integral to their work when using Counselling Skills.

continued . . .

Code of Ethics & Practice

1 January 1999

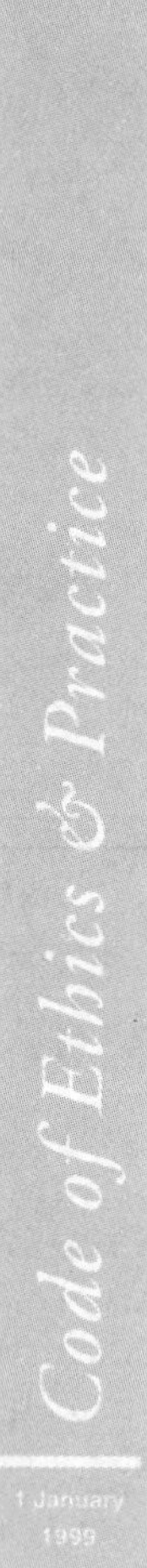

C.3 Confidentiality

C.3.1 Practitioners offer the highest possible levels of confidentiality consistent with their primary professional or work role.

C.3.2 Any limits to confidentiality must be made explicit.

C.4 Competence

C.4.1 Practitioners are responsible for ensuring that they have training in the use of Counselling Skills and that this training is appropriate and sufficient for the Counselling Skills work they undertake.

C.4.2 Practitioners are responsible for working within the limits of their competence.

C.4.3 Both practitioners and the organisations for whom they work have a responsibility for monitoring and developing the practitioner's competence in the use of Counselling Skills. Non-managerial supervision is recognised as one of the best methods for achieving this.

C.4.4 Both practitioners and their organisations have a responsibility for addressing those aspects of an organisation which impede the ethical use of Counselling Skills.

C.5 Integration of Codes of Ethics and Practice

Many of those who use Counselling Skills in their work are also bound by another Code of Ethics and Practice relating to their primary professional or work role. Practitioners therefore have responsibility for managing the integration of this Code with any other Code and for resolving difficulties or conflicts which may arise. It is important to recognise any way in which the primary role limits the use of Counselling Skills.

D. *Practice Guidelines*

These guidelines apply the values and ethical principles outlined in this Code of Ethics for use in practice. Within another role the Counselling Skills user may help someone to recognise feelings, thoughts and behaviours and, when appropriate, to explore them in greater depth. The guidelines address issues of competence relating to these skills in practice.

D.1 Confidentiality

Confidentiality is crucial to the working relationship. For this reason any limits to the degree of confidentiality offered must be carefully considered. As the use of Counselling Skills often takes place within a network of overlapping accountabilities the following clauses need to be understood within the context of the network.

Practitioners must therefore:

D.1.1 have clarified for themselves the extent of confidentiality which is consistent with any other roles they hold whilst using Counselling Skills

D.1.2 when appropriate, reach an agreement with the client at the outset about the extent of confidentiality

D.1.3 take great care not to disclose, either inadvertently or under pressure, information given in confidence

D.1.4 wherever possible, negotiate any change in the agreement with the client.

D.1.5 ensure confidentiality of material relating to the use of Counselling Skills which is used either for research purposes or in presenting cases for supervision or training.

Practitioners using such material must therefore:

D.1.6 where appropriate, obtain the consent of the client for such use

D.1.7 effectively disguise the client's identity

continued . . .

D.1.8 ensure that discussion about such material is respectful and purposeful and is not trivialising.

D.2 Competent Practice

Practitioners should consider:

D.2.1 whether it is appropriate to use Counselling Skills within their other role

D.2.2 whether their level of training in the use of Counselling Skills is adequate for the work in each individual instance or setting

D.2.3 how any other relevant professional Codes might affect their use of Counselling Skills within the work and whether any specific limits to confidentiality arise

D.2.4 how any emerging areas of potential role conflict could be resolved

D.2.5 whether the purpose of using Counselling Skills within a given context is clear to the client

D.2.6 whether the necessary arrangements have been made with colleagues to ensure that an environment offering safety and privacy can be provided

D.2.7 the power aspect of relationships within the work and any consequent need to address this

D.2.8 the significance of their own and the client's social and cultural contexts in the work undertaken

D.2.9 establishing an appropriate referral network

and should:

D.2.10 value and facilitate the expression of thoughts and feelings

D.2.11 acknowledge the client's thoughts and feelings and consider whether further exploration is appropriate or not at that moment

D.2.12 be aware of their responsibility to resolve conflicts between ethical priorities

D.2.13 be respectful of the client's world

D.2.14 ensure non-discriminatory practice in their Counselling Skills work

D.2.15 recognise when it is appropriate to refer a client elsewhere

D.2.16 recognise and work with the client's reactions to the referral process

D.2.17 wherever possible, make an appropriate closure of any Counselling Skills work

D.2.18 consider any responsibilities there may be for follow up.

D.3 Supervision

Regular and formalised non-managerial supervision for practitioners is widely recognised as good practice and is highly recommended. It should be an adjunct to managerial supervision of the total work.

Supervision offers practitioners a regular opportunity, outside the line management system, to discuss and monitor their Counselling Skills work whilst still maintaining client confidentiality. It is a formal, collaborative process which is primarily concerned with the well being of the client and secondarily with that of the practitioner

The supervisor will have knowledge and experience in using Counselling Skills and will also be familiar with the Code of Ethics and Practice.

Supervision can:

- help practitioners to maintain ethical and professional standards of practice
- enhance confidence, clarity and competence in the work

continued . . .

BRITISH ASSOCIATION FOR COUNSELLING

Code of Ethics & Practice

1 January 1999

- develop constructive thinking about the effectiveness of the work
- acknowledge and help to recognise and manage the emotional impact of the work in order to enhance effectiveness and prevent burnout

Further guidance on the ethics and practice of supervision can be obtained from BAC's Code of Ethics and Practice for Supervisors.

D.4 Accountability

Practitioners are accountable for their work to the client, the organisations in which they may practise and their professional bodies.

Practitioners should therefore:

D.4.1 have received adequate basic training

D.4.2 maintain ongoing skills development and relevant learning

D.4.3 monitor their personal functioning and seek help or withdraw from using Counselling Skills, temporarily or permanently, if their personal resources become sufficiently depleted to require this

D.4.4 take all reasonable steps to ensure their own safety

D.4.5 evaluate their practice, drawing where appropriate on feedback from clients, colleagues and managers

D.4.6 recognise the impact of their own beliefs and prejudices on the work they do

D.4.7 monitor their work to ensure that they are not discriminating against or disadvantaging their clients

D.4.8 exercise caution before engaging in a different type of relationship with those who are or have been clients (e.g. to a business, social, sexual, training, therapeutic or other relationship) and consult with a supervisor or manager whether such a change is appropriate.

Equal Opportunities Policy Statement

'The British Association for Counselling' (BAC) is committed to promoting Equality of Opportunity of access and participation for all its members in all of its structures and their workings. BAC has due regard for those groups of people with identifiable characteristics which can lead to visible and invisible barriers thus inhibiting their joining and full participation in BAC. Barriers can include age, colour, creed, culture, disability, education, ethnicity, gender, information, knowledge, mobility, money, nationality, race, religion, sexual orientation, social class and status.

The work of BAC aims to reflect this commitment in all areas including services to members, employer responsibilities, the recruitment of and working with volunteers, setting, assessing, monitoring and evaluating standards and the implementation of the complaints procedures. This is particularly important as BAC is the 'Voice of Counselling' in the wider world.

BAC will promote and encourage commitment to Equality of Opportunity by its members.

 4 Effective from 1 January 1999

Code of Ethics & Practice

1 January 1996

For Supervisors of Counsellors

1. Status of the Code

1.1 In response to the experience of members of BAC, this Code is a revision of the 1988 Code of Ethics & Practice for the Supervision of Counsellors.

2. Introduction

2.1 The purpose of the Code is to establish and maintain standards for supervisors who are members of BAC and to inform and protect counsellors seeking supervision. Throughout this Code the terms Counsellor and Counselling are used in accordance with the definition of counselling in the Code of Ethics & Practice for Counsellors.

2.2 All members of this Association are required to abide by existing Codes appropriate to them. They thereby accept a common frame of reference within which to manage their responsibilities to supervisees and their clients, colleagues, members of this Association and the wider community. Whilst this Code cannot resolve all ethical and practice related issues, it aims to provide a framework for addressing ethical issues and to encourage optimum levels of practice. Supervisors and supervisees (counsellors) will need to judge which parts of this Code apply to particular situations They may have to decide between conflicting responsibilities.

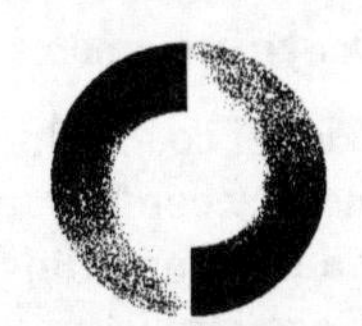

British Association for Counselling
1 Regent Place • Rugby • Warwickshire CV21 2PJ
Tel 01788 550899 • Fax 01788 562189 • Minicom 01788 572838 • e-mail bac@bac.co.uk
Company limited by guarantee 2175320 registered in England & Wales • Registered Charity 298361

2.3 Counselling Supervision is a formal and mutually agreed arrangement for counsellors to discuss their work regularly with someone who is normally an experienced and competent counsellor and familiar with the process of counselling supervision. The task is to work together to ensure and develop the efficacy of the supervisee's counselling practice.

Counselling Supervision is the term that will be used throughout this Code. It is also known as supervision, consultative support, clinical supervision or non-managerial supervision. It is an essential part of good practice for counselling. It is different from training, personal development and line management accountability.

2.4 This Association has a Complaints Procedure which can lead to the expulsion of members for breaches of its Codes of Ethics & Practice.

3. Nature of Counselling Supervision

3.1 Counselling supervision provides supervisees with the opportunity on a regular basis to discuss and monitor their work with clients. It should take account of the setting in which supervisees practise. Counselling supervision is intended to ensure that the needs of the clients are being addressed and to monitor the effectiveness of the therapeutic interventions.

3.2 Counselling supervision may contain some elements of training, personal development or line-management, but counselling supervision is not primarily intended for these purposes and appropriate management of these issues should be observed.

3.3 Counselling supervision is a formal collaborative process intended to help supervisees maintain ethical and professional standards of practice and to enhance creativity.

3.4 It is essential that counsellor and supervisor are able to work together constructively as counselling supervision includes supportive and challenging elements.

3.5 There are several modes of counselling supervision (see 5), which vary in appropriateness according to the needs of supervisees. More than one mode of counselling supervision may be used concurrently. This Code applies to all counselling supervision arrangements.

3.6 The frequency of counselling supervision will vary according to the volume of counselling, the experience of supervisees and their work setting.

4. Anti-discriminatory Practice in Counselling Supervision

4.1 Anti-discriminatory practice underpins the basic values of counselling and counselling supervision as stated in this document and in the Code of Ethics & Practice for Counsellors. It also addresses the issue of the client's social context, B.2.7.3 of that Code (1996).

4.2 Supervisors have a responsibility to be aware of their own issues of prejudice and stereotyping, and particularly to consider ways in which this may be affecting the supervisory relationship. Discussion of this is part of the counselling supervision process.

4.3 Supervisors need to be alert to any prejudices and assumptions that counsellors reveal in their work with clients and to raise awareness of these so that the needs of clients may be met with more sensitivity. One purpose of counselling supervision is to enable supervisees to recognise and value difference. Supervisors have a responsibility to challenge the appropriateness of the work of a supervisee whose own belief system interferes with the acceptance of clients.

4.4 Attitudes, assumptions and prejudices can be identified by the language used, and by paying attention to the selectivity of material brought to counselling supervision.

5. Modes of Counselling Supervision

There are different modes of counselling supervision. The particular features of some of these modes are outlined below. Some counsellors use combinations of these for their counselling supervision.

5.1 **One to One, Supervisor-Supervisee**

This involves a supervisor providing counselling supervision on an individual basis for an individual counsellor who is usually less experienced than the supervisor. This is the most widely used mode of counselling supervision.

5.2 **Group Counselling Supervision with Identified Counselling Supervisor(s)**

There are several ways of providing this form of counselling supervision. In one approach the supervisor acts as the leader, takes responsibility for organising the time equally between the supervisees, and concentrates on the work of each individual in turn. Using another approach the supervisees allocate counselling supervision time between themselves with the supervisor as a technical resource.

5.3 **One to One Peer Counselling Supervision**

This involves two participants providing counselling supervision for each other by alternating the roles of supervisor and supervisee. Typically, the time available for counselling supervision is divided equally between them. This mode on its own is not suitable for all practitioners.

5.4 **Peer Group Counselling Supervision**

This takes place when three or more counsellors share the responsibility for providing each other's counselling supervision within the group. Typically, they will consider themselves to be of broadly equal status, training and/or experience. This mode on its own is unsuitable for inexperienced practitioners.

5.5 Particular issues of competence for each mode are detailed in the Code of Practice B.2.6.

6 The Structure of this Code

6.1 This Code has two sections. Section A, the Code of Ethics, outlines the fundamental values of counselling supervision and a number of general principles arising from these. Section B, the Code of Practice, applies these principles to counselling supervision.

A CODE OF ETHICS

A.1 Counselling supervision is a non-exploitative activity. Its basic values are integrity, responsibility, impartiality and respect. Supervisors must take the same degree of care to work ethically whether they are paid or work voluntarily and irrespective of the mode of counselling supervision used.

A.2 Confidentiality

The content of counselling supervision is highly confidential. Supervisors must clarify their limits of confidentiality.

A.3 Safety

All reasonable steps must be taken to ensure the safety of supervisees and their clients during their work together.

A.4 Effectiveness

All reasonable steps must be taken by supervisors to encourage optimum levels of practice by supervisees.

A.5 Contracts

The terms and conditions on which counselling supervision is offered must be made clear to supervisees at the outset. Subsequent revisions of these terms must be agreed in advance of any change.

A.6 Competence

Supervisors must take all reasonable steps to monitor and develop their own competence and to work within the limits of that competence. This includes having supervision of their supervision work.

B CODE OF PRACTICE

B.1 Issues of Responsibility

B.1.1 Supervisors are responsible for ensuring that an individual contract is worked out with their supervisees which will allow them to present and explore their work as honestly as possible.

B.1.2 Within this contract supervisors are responsible for helping supervisees to reflect critically upon their work, while at the same time acknowledging that clinical responsibility remains with the counsellor.

B.1.3 Supervisors are responsible, together with their supervisees, for ensuring that the best use is made of counselling supervision time, in order to address the needs of clients.

B.1.4 Supervisors are responsible for setting and maintaining the boundaries between the counselling supervision relationship and other professional relationships, e.g. training and management.

B.1.5 Supervisors and supervisees should take all reasonable steps to ensure that any personal or social contact between them does not adversely influence the effectiveness of the counselling supervision.

B.1.6 A supervisor must not have a counselling supervision and a personal counselling contract with the same supervisee over the same period of time.

B.1.7 Supervisors must not exploit their supervisees financially, sexually, emotionally or in any other way. It is unethical for supervisors to engage in sexual activity with their supervisee.

B.1.8 Supervisors have a responsibility to enquire about any other relationships which may exist between supervisees and their clients as these may impair the objectivity and professional judgement of supervisees.

B.1.9 Supervisors must recognise, and work in ways that respects the value and dignity of supervisees and their clients with due regard to issues such as origin, status, race, gender, age, beliefs, sexual orientation and disability. This must include raising awareness of any discriminatory practices that may exist between supervisees and their clients, or between supervisor and supervisee.

B.1.10 Supervisors must ensure that together with their supervisees they consider their respective legal liabilities to each other, to the employing or training organisation, if any, and to clients.

B.1.11 Supervisors are responsible for taking actionif they are aware that their supervisees' practice is not in accordance with BAC's Codes of Ethics & Practice for Counsellors.

B.1.12 Supervisors are responsible for helping their supervisees recognise when their functioning as counsellors is impaired due to personal or emotional difficulties, any condition that affects judgement, illness, the influence of alcohol or drugs, or for any other reason, and for ensuring that appropriate action is taken.

B.1.13 Supervisors must conduct themselves in their supervision-related activities in ways which do not undermine public confidence in either their role as a supervisor or in the work of other supervisors.

B.1.14 If a supervisor is aware of possible misconduct by another supervisor which cannot be resolved or remedied after discussion with the supervisor concerned, they should implement the Complaints Procedure, doing so within the boundaries of confidentiality required by the Complaints Procedure.

B.1.15 Supervisors are responsible for ensuring that their emotional needs are met outside the counselling supervision work and are not solely dependent on their relationship with supervisees.

B.1.16 Supervisors are responsible for consulting with their own supervisor before former clients are taken on as supervisees or former supervisees are taken on as clients.

B.2 Issues of Competence

B.2.1 Under all of the modes of counselling supervision listed above, supervisors should normally be practising and experienced counsellors.

B.2.2 Supervisors are responsible for seeking ways to further their own professional development.

B.2.3 Supervisors are responsible for making arrangements for their own supervision in order to support their counselling supervision work and to help them to evaluate their competence.

B.2.4 Supervisors are responsible for monitoring and working within the limits of their competence.

B.2.5 Supervisors are responsible for withdrawing from counselling supervision work either temporarily or permanently when their functioning is impaired due to personal or emotional difficulties, illness, the influence of alcohol or drugs, or for any other reason.

B.2.6 Some modes require extra consideration and these are detailed in this section.

	A	B	C	D	E	F	G	H
One to one supervisor-supervisee	X							
Group counselling supervision with identified and more experienced supervisor	X	X		X	X			
One to one peer counselling supervision	X	X	X	X			X	X
Peer group counselling supervision	X	X	X	X		X	X	X

A. All points contained elsewhere within the Code of Practice should be considered.

B. Sufficient time must be allocated to each counsellor to ensure adequate supervision of their counselling work.

C. This method on its own is particularly unsuitable for trainees, recently trained or inexperienced counsellors.

D. Care needs to be taken to develop an atmosphere conducive to sharing, questioning and challenging each others' practice in a constructive and supportive way.

E. As well as having a background in counselling work, supervisors should have appropriate groupwork experience in order to facilitate this kind of group.

F. All participants should have sufficient groupwork experience to be able to engage the group process in ways which facilitate effective counselling supervision.

G. Explicit consideration should be given to deciding who is responsible for providing the counselling supervision, and how the task of counselling supervision will be carried out.

H. It is good practice to have an independent consultant to visit regularly to observe and monitor the process and quality of the counselling supervision.

B.3 Management of Work

B.3.1 The Counselling Supervision Contract

3.1.1 Where supervisors and supervisees work for the same agency or organisation the supervisor is responsible for clarifying all contractual obligations.

3.1.2 Supervisors must inform their supervisee, as appropriate, about their own training, philosophy and theoretical position, qualifications, approach to anti-discriminatory practice and the methods of counselling supervision they use.

3.1.3 Supervisors must be explicit regarding practical arrangements for counselling supervision, paying particular regard to the length of contact time, the frequency of contact, policy and practice regarding record keeping, and the privacy of the venue.

3.1.4 Fees and fee increases must be arranged and agreed in advance.

3.1.5 Supervisors and supervisees must make explicit the expectations and requirements they have of each other. This should include the manner in which any formal assessment of the supervisee's work will be conducted. Each party should assess the value of working with the other, and review this regularly.

3.1.6 Supervisors must discuss their policy regarding giving references and any fees that may be charged for this or for any other work done outside counselling supervision time.

3.1.7 Before formalising a counselling supervision contract supervisors must ascertain what personal counselling the supervisee has or has had. This is in order to take into account any effect this may have on the supervisee's counselling work.

3.1.8 Supervisors working with trainee counsellors must clarify the boundaries of their responsibility and their accountability to their supervisee and to the training course and any agency/placement involved. This should include any formal assessment required.

B.3.2 Confidentiality

3.2.1 As a general principle, supervisors must not reveal confidential material concerning the supervisee or their clients to any other person without the express consent of all parties concerned. Exceptions to this general principle are contained within this Code.

3.2.2 When initial contracts are being made, agreements about the people to whom supervisors may speak about their supervisees work must include those on whom the supervisors rely for support, supervision or consultancy. There must also be clarity at this stage about the boundaries of confidentiality having regard for the supervisor's own framework of accountability. This is particularly relevant when providing counselling supervision to a trainee counsellor.

3.2.3 Supervisors should take all reasonable steps to encourage supervisees to present their work in ways which protect the personal identity of clients, or to get their client's informed consent to present information which could lead to personal identification.

3.2.4 Supervisors must not reveal confidential information concerning supervisees or their clients to any person or through any public medium except:

a. When it is clearly stated in the counselling supervision contract and it is in accordance with all BAC Codes of Ethics & Practice.

b. When the supervisor considers it necessary to prevent serious emotional or physical damage to the client, the supervisee or a third party. In such circumstances the supervisee's consent to a change in the agreement about confidentiality should be sought, unless there are good grounds for believing that the supervisee is no longer able to take responsibility for his/her own actions. Whenever possible, the decision to break confidentiality in any circumstances should be made after consultation with another experienced supervisor.

3.2.5 The disclosure of confidential information relating to supervisees is permissible when relevant to the following situations:

a. Recommendations concerning supervisees for professional purposes e.g. references and assessments.

b. Pursuit of disciplinary action involving supervisees in matters pertaining to standards of ethics and practice.

In the latter instance, any breaking of confidentiality should be minimised by conveying only information pertinent to the immediate situation on a need-to-know basis. The ethical considerations needing to be taken into account are:

i. Maintaining the best interests of the supervisee

ii. Enabling the supervisee to take responsibility for their actions

iii. Taking full account of the supervisor's responsibility to the client and to the wider community

3.2.6 Information about work with a supervisee may be used for publication or in meetings only with the supervisee's permission and with anonymity preserved.

3.2.7 On occasions when it is necessary to consult with professional colleagues, supervisors ensure that their discussion is purposeful and not trivialising.

B.3.3 The Management of Counselling Supervision

3.3.1 Supervisors must encourage the supervisee to belong to an association or organisation with a Code of Ethics & Practice and a Complaints Procedure. This provides additional safeguards for the supervisor, supervisee and client in the event of a complaint.

3.3.2 If, in the course of counselling supervision, it appears that personal counselling may be necessary for the supervisee to be able to continue working effectively, the supervisor should raise this issue with the supervisee.

3.3.3 Supervisors must monitor regularly how their supervisees engage in self-assessment and the self-evaluation of their work.

3.3.4 Supervisors must ensure that their supervisees acknowledge their individual responsibility for ongoing professional development and for participating in further training programmes.

3.3.5 Supervisors must ensure that their supervisees are aware of the distinction between counselling, accountability to management, counselling supervision and training.

3.3.6 Supervisors must ensure with a supervisee who works in an organisation or agency that the lines of accountability and responsibility are clearly defined: supervisee/client; supervisor/supervisee; supervisor/client; organisation/supervisor; organisation/supervisee; organisation/client. There is a distinction between line management supervision and counselling supervision.

3.3.7 Best practice is that the same person should not act as both line manager and counselling supervisor to the same supervisee. However, where the counselling supervisor is also the line manager, the supervisee should have access to independent counselling supervision.

3.3.8 Supervisors who become aware of a conflict between an obligation to a supervisee and an obligation to an employing agency must make explicit to the supervisee the nature of the loyalties and responsibilities involved.

3.3.9 Supervisors who have concerns about a supervisee's work with clients must be clear how they will pursue this if discussion in counselling supervision fails to resolve the situation.

3.3.10 Where disagreements cannot be resolved by discussions between supervisor and supervisee, the supervisor should consult with a fellow professional and, if appropriate, recommend that the supervisee be referred to another supervisor.

3.3.11 Supervisors must discuss with supervisees the need to have arrangements in place to take care of the immediate needs of clients in the event of a sudden and unplanned ending to the counselling relationship. It is good practice forthe supervisor to be informed about these arrangements.

 AGM Sept 1995 • Effective 1 Jan 1996

Recommended reading

Bayne, R., Horton, I. and Bimrose, J. (1996) *New Directions in Counselling*, Routledge, London.

A range of issues are addressed here: the impact of accreditation, National Vocational Qualifications, developing codes of ethics and evaluating effectiveness. All in all, a useful book for anyone who wants to keep up to date with their reading about counselling.

Berg, R.C., Landreth, G.L. and Fall, K.A. (1998) *Group Counselling: Concepts and Procedures*, 3rd edn, Taylor and Francis, London.

This new edition provides a thorough discussion of the rationale for using group counselling and offers practical suggestions on the skills needed to run therapeutic groups.

Burnard, P. (1996) *Acquiring Interpersonal Skills: a Handbook of Experiential Learning for Health Professionals*, 2nd edn, Stanley Thornes, Cheltenham.

In this book, I have offered a theoretical review of experiential learning – or learning from personal experience – and show how theory and research can be put into practice in the teaching of interpersonal skills.

Crompton, M. (1992) *Children and Counselling*, Edward Arnold, London.

This is a very warm and human account of ways in which counsellors might work with children. Margaret Crompton sensitively and practically tackles a series of timely issues in this engaging book.

Crouch, A. (1997) *Inside Counselling: Becoming and Being a Professional Counsellor*, Sage, London.

This is a first-person account, by the author, of what it is like to be a counsellor. This is something of a 'one-off' and the first-person style may not appeal to all readers, although the book offers some important insights into what it is like to practise counselling.

East, P. (1995) *Counselling Skills in Medical Settings*, Open University Press, Buckingham.

Another practical book in which the author draws examples from medical practice and discusses issues relating to change and the delivery of health and community care.

Goldberg, D. and Huxley, P. (1992) *Common Mental Disorders: a bio-social model*, Routledge, London.

A scholarly and extremely well-referenced book that will be useful for those who want to expand their knowledge of mental illness.

Hammersley, D. (1995) *Counselling People on Prescribed Drugs*, Sage, London.

A very practical book which will be of value to anyone who works with those who are taking drugs or withdrawing from them. The author also explores the complex problems of overdosing, psychotic episodes and antisocial behaviour.

Heron, J. (1989) *The Facilitators' Handbook*, Kogan Page, London.

A classic text in which Heron, a leading humanistic trainer and philosopher, outlines his approach to teaching and training in interpersonal skills and counselling.

Hough, M. (1998) *Counselling Skills and Theory*, Hodder and Stoughton, London.

This is perhaps more about theory than skills but it offers a very readable account of the psychodynamic, person-centred, gestalt, transactional analysis, behavioural and cognitive approaches to counselling.

McLoughlin, B. (1995) *Developing Psychodynamic Counselling*, Sage, London.

McLoughlin offers a very useful and specific account of one approach to counselling. The book contains plenty of case examples and points for discussion.

Nelson-Jones, R. (1995) *The Theory and Practice of Counselling*, 2nd edn, Cassell, London.

This is a thoroughly revised and updated version of Nelson-Jones' standard and excellent text, *The Theory and Practice of Counselling Psychology*. In an easy-to-read style, Nelson-Jones offers a detailed exploration of all the various and current approaches to counselling. This is a detailed textbook, ideal for students on counselling courses.

O'Leary, E. (1995) *Counselling Older Adults: Perspectives, Approaches and Research*, Stanley Thornes, Cheltenham.

This book offers a consideration of the theory and application of general counselling approaches to this increasing and important section of society. Case studies and counselling transcripts are included.

Palmer, S. and McMahon, G. (1997) *Handbook of Counselling*, 2nd edn, Routledge, London.

All the contributors to this large book are experienced practitioners and the book offers a comprehensive series of essays about a huge range of areas to do with counselling. A useful book for student counsellors.

Palmer, S., Dainow, S. and Milner, P. (1996) *Counselling: the BAC Counselling Reader*, Sage, London, in association with the British Association for Counselling.

This book offers articles previously published in *Counselling*, the journal of the British Association for Counselling. It is likely to be useful to those who are new to counselling and who want to explore what contributors to *Counselling* have to say about the subject. A comprehensive book.

Rogers, C.R. (1951) *Client-Centred Therapy*, Constable, London.

The book in which Rogers describes much of the research that led him to adopt the client centred way of working in counselling and therapy. Certainly not as easy to read as *On Becoming a Person* but an important book for those interested in the history of counselling.

Rogers, C.R. (1967) *On Becoming a Person: a Therapist's View of Psychotherapy*, Constable, London.

A classic text that is essential reading for anyone interested in the client centred approach to counselling. Rogers had an easy-to-read style that made his work immediately accessible to a wide range of readers. This book is a series of essays and is still in print.

Stewart, W. (1997) *A–Z of Counselling Theory and Practice*, 2nd edn, Stanley Thornes, Cheltenham.

A rather idiosyncratic book that is not always clearly referenced but which does offer a user-friendly approach to looking up key concepts.

Stoter, D. (1995) *Spiritual Aspects of Health Care*, Mosby, London.

A useful book for those who want to think more about their clients' and patients' spiritual needs.

Thompson, R. A. (1996) *Counselling Techniques: Improving Relationships with others, our Families and our Environment*, Taylor and Francis, London.

This book provides counselling techniques from a broad range of theoretical approaches and is particularly strong on the issue of clients taking on an increased responsibility for themselves in the counselling process.

Wheeler, S. (1996) *Training Counsellors: the Assessment of Competence*, Cassell, London.

This is a very practical book for those who want to run counselling courses. It pays particular attention to assessing counselling competence – a topic not regularly addressed in the literature.

Wiger, D. E. (1999) *The Psychotherapy Documentation Primer*, Wiley, New York.

This will be useful to anyone who is confused about how to record their counselling sessions.

Wondrak, R. (1998) *Interpersonal Skills for Nurses and Health Care Professionals*, Blackwell, Oxford.

The author offers a 'lifespan' approach to thinking about interpersonal skills and discusses some of the theories underlying skilled interpersonal practice.

References

Alberti, R.E. and Emmons, M.L. (1982) *Your Perfect Right: a Guide to Assertive Living*, 4th edn, Impact Publishers, San Luis, California.

Alexander, F.M. (1969) *Resurrection of the Body*, University Books, New York.

Andersen, H. and MacElveen-Hoen, P. (1988) Gay clients with AIDS: new challenges for hospice programs. *Hospice Journal: Physical, Psychosocial and Pastoral Care of the Dying*, **4**(2), 37–54.

Argyle, M. (1975) *The Psychology of Interpersonal Behaviour*, Penguin, Harmondsworth.

Ashton, J. and Seymour, H.J. (1988) *The New Public Health*, Open University Press, Milton Keynes.

Ball, B. (1984) *Careers Counselling in Practice*, Falmer Press, London.

Bancroft, J. (1983) *Human Sexuality and its Problems*, Churchill Livingstone, Edinburgh.

Bandler, R. and Grinder, J. (1975) *The Stucture of Magic, Volume I: a Book About Language and Therapy*, Science and Behavior Books, California.

Bandler, R. and Grinder, J. (1982) *Reframing: Neuro-Linguistic Programming and the Transformation of Meaning*, Real People Press, Moab, Utah.

Bannister, D. and Fransella, F. (1986) *Inquiring Man*, 2nd edn, Penguin, Harmondsworth.

Barnett, R. (1994) *The Limits of Competence*, SRHE and Open University Press, Buckingham.

Barrett-Lennard, G.T. (1981) The empathy cycle – refinement of a nuclear concept. *Journal of Counselling Psychology*, **28**, 91–100.

Barrett-Lennard. G.T. (1993) The phases and focus of empathy. *British Journal of Medical Psychology*, **66**, 3–14.

Beane, J. (1981) 'I'd rather be dead than gay: counselling gay men who are coming out.' *Personnel and Guidance Journal*, **60**(4), 222–6.

Beck, A., Rush, A., Shaw, B. and Emery, C. (1979) *Cognitive Therapy of Depression*, Wiley, Chichester.

Berne, E. (1964) *Games People Play*, Penguin, Harmondsworth.

Berne, E. (1972) *What Do You Say After You Say Hello*? Corgi, London.

Bor, R. (1991) The ABC of AIDS counselling. *Nursing Times*, **87**(1), 32–35.

Bor, R., Miller, R., Perry, L. *et al.* (1989) Strategies for counselling the 'worried well' in relation to AIDS. *Journal of the Royal Society of Medicine*, **23**, 218–20.

Bowen, D. (1990) *Shaking the Iron Universe*, Hodder and Stoughton, London.

Bowlby, J. (1975) *Separation*, Penguin, Harmondsworth.

Bradshaw, A. (1997) Teaching spiritual care to nurses: an alternative approach. *International Journal of Palliative Nursing*, **3**(1), 51–7.

Brandes, D. and Phillips, R. (1984) *The Gamester's Handbook*, Vol 2, Hutchinson, London.

British Association for Counselling (BAC) (1989a) *Invitation to Membership*, BAC, Rugby.

British Association for Counselling (BAC) (1989b) *Code of Ethics and Practice for Counselling Skills*, BAC, Rugby.

Brown, R. (1986) *Social Psychology*, 3rd edn, Collier Macmillan, New York.

Buber, M. (1948) *Tales of Hasidism: the Later Masters*, Schocken, New York.
Buber, M. (1958) *I and Thou*, 2nd edn, Scribner, New York.
Buber, M. (1966) *The Knowledge of Man: a Philosophy of the Interhuman.* (ed. M Freidman, trans.) R.G. Smith, Harper and Row, New York.
Bugental, E.K. and Bugental, J.F.T. (1984) Dispiritedness: a new perspective on a familiar state. *Journal of Humanistic Psychology* 24, 49–67.
Bugental, J.F.T. (1980) The far side of despair. *Journal of Humanistic Psychology*, 20 49–68.
Burnard, P. (1985) *Learning Human Skills*, Heinemann, London.
Burnard, P. (1995) *Counselling Skills for Health Professionals*, 2nd edn, Chapman and Hall, London.
Burnard, P. (1996) *Acquiring Interpersonal Skills: a Handbook of Experiential Learning for Health Professionals*, 2nd edn, Stanley Thornes, Cheltenham.
Burnard, P. (1997) *Effective Communication Skills for Health Professionals*, 2nd edn, Stanley Thornes, Cheltenham.
Burnard, P. and Morrison, P. (1987) Nurses' perceptions of their interpersonal skills, *Nursing Times*, 82(43), 59.
Calnan, J. (1983) *Talking With Patients*, Heinemann, London.
Campbell, A. (1984a) *Paid to Care?* SPCK, London.
Campbell, A. (1984b) *Moderated Love*, SPCK, London.
Carkuff, R.R. (1969) *Helping and Human Relations, Volume 1: Selection and Training*, Holt, Rinehart and Winston, New York.
Chapman, A.J. and Gale, A. (1982) *Psychology and People: a Tutorial Text*, British Psychological Society and Macmillan, London.
Claxton, G. (1984) *Live and Learn: an Introduction to the Psychology of Growth and Change in Everday Life*, Harper and Row, London.
Clift, J.C. and Imrie, B.W. (1981) *Assessing Students, Appraising Teaching*, Croom Helm, London.
Coles, R. (1992) *The Spiritual Life of Children*, Harper Collins, London.
Coltart, N. (1993) *How to Survive as a Psychotherapist*, Sheldon Press, London.
Connor, S. and Kingman, S. (1989) *The Search for the Virus: the Scientific Discovery of AIDS and the Quest for a Cure*, Penguin, Harmondsworth.
Cook, A., Fischer, G., Jones, E. *et al.* (1988) *Preventing AIDS Among Substance Abusers: a Training Manual for Substance Abuse Treatment Counsellors*, The Center for AIDS and Substance Abuse Training, Falls Church, VA.
Cox, M. (1978) *Structuring the Therapeutic Process*, Pergamon Press, London.
Crowley, J. (1997) Education: therapeutic teaching and the education of student midwives, *British Journal of Midwifery*, 5(3), 159–62.
Crystal, D. (1987) *The Cambridge Encyclopedia of Language*, Cambridge University Press, Cambridge.
Davies, D. (1987) *Counselling in Psychological Settings*, Open University Press, Buckingham.
Davis, H. and Fallowfield, L. (eds) (1991a) *Counselling and Communication in Health Care*, Wiley, Chichester.
Dennis, H. (1991) Getting the Message. *Nursing Standard*, 5(17), 55–6.
Dewey, J. (1966) *Democracy and Education*, Free Press, London.
Dewey, J. (1971) *Experience and Education*, Collier Macmillan, London.
Dilley, J.W., Pies, C. and Helquist, M. (1989) *Face to Face: a guide to AIDS counselling*, AIDS Health Project, University of California, San Francisco, California.
DiMarzo, D. (1989) Double jeopardy: haemophilia and HIV disease. *AIDS Care*, 1, 51–8.

DiScenza, S., Nies, M. and Jordan, C. (1996) Effectiveness of counselling in the health promotion of HIV positive clients in the community. *Public Health Nursing*, 13(3), 209–16.

Dorn, F.J. (ed.) (1986) *The Social Influence Process in Counselling and Psychotherapy*, Thomas, Springfield, Illinois.

Dryden, W., Charles-Edwards, D. and Woolfe, R. (eds) (1989) *Handbook of Counselling in Britain*, Routledge, London.

Dryden, W., Horton, I. and Mearns, D. (1995) *Issues in Professional Counsellor Training*, Cassell, London.

D'Zurilla, T.J. and Goldfried, M.R. (1971) Problem solving and behavior modification. *Journal of Abnormal Psychology*, 78, 107–26.

Egan, G. (1982) *The Skilled Helper*, 2nd edn, Brooks/Cole, Monterey, California.

Egan, G. (1990) *The Skilled Helper: a Systematic Approach to Effective Helping*, 5th edition, Brooks/Cole, Monterey, California.

Ellis, A. (1962) *Reason and Emotion in Psychotherapy*, Lyle, Stuart, New Jersey.

Ellis, A. (1987) The evolution of rational-emotive therapy (RET) and cognitive behaviour therapy (CBT). In: J.K. Zeig (ed.) *The Evolution of Psychotherapy*, Brunner/Mazel, New York.

Ellis, A. and Dryden, W. (1987) *The Practice of Rational-Emotive Therapy*, Springer, New York.

Ellis, R. and McClintock, A. (1994) *If You Take My Meaning: Theory into Practice in Human Communication*, 2nd edn, Edward Arnold, London.

ENB (1982) *Syllabus of Training: Professional Register – Part 3: (Registered Mental Nurse)*, English and Welsh National Boards for Nursing, Midwifery and Health Visiting, London and Cardiff.

Epting, T.R. (1984) *Personal Construct Counselling and Psychotherapy*, Wiley, Chichester.

Erikson, E. (1959) *Identity and the Life Cycle*, International Universities Press, New York.

Ernst, S. and Goodison, L. (1981) *In Our Own Hands: a Book of Self-Help Therapy*, Women's Press, London.

Fairburn, C.G., Dickerson, M.G. and Greenwood, J. (1983) *Sexual Problems and their Management*, Churchill Livingstone, Edinburgh.

Faltz, B.G. (1989) Strategies for working with substance abusing clients. In: J.W. Dilley, C. Pies and M. Helquist, (eds) *Face to Face: a Guide to AIDS Counselling*, AIDS Health Project, University of California, San Francisco.

Farrelly, F. and Brandsma, J. (1974) *Provocative Therapy*, Meta, Cupertino, California.

Faulkner, A., Webb, P. and Maquire, P. (1991) Communication and counselling skills: educating health professionals working in cancer and palliative care. *Patient Education and Counselling*, 18(1), 3–7.

Fay, A. (1978) *Making Things Better by Making Them Worse*, Hawthorne, New York.

Fay, A. (1986) Clinical notes on paradoxical thearpy. *Psychotherapy: Theory, Research and Practice*, 18(1), 14–22.

Feldenkrais, M. (1972) *Awareness Through Movement*, Harper and Row, New York.

Feltham, C. and Dryden, W. (1993) *Dictionary of Counselling*, Whurr, London.

Ferguson, E. (1998) Once more – with feeling. *The Observer*, 30th August.

Fiedler, F. E. (1950) The concept of an ideal therapeutic relationship. *Journal of Consulting Psychology*, 14 239–45.

Fordham, F. (1966) *An Introduction to Jung's Psychology*, Penguin, Harmondsworth.

Frankl, V.E. (1959) *Man's Search for Meaning*, Beacon Press, New York.

Frankl, V.E. (1960) Paradoxical intention: a logotherapeutic technique. *American Journal of Psychotherapy* **14**, 520–35.

Frankl, V.E. (1969) *The Will to Meaning*, World Publishing, New York.

Frankl, V.E. (1975) *The Unconscious God*, Simon and Schuster, New York.

Fullilove, M.T. (1989) Ethnic minorities, HIV disease and the growing underclass. In: J.W. Dilley, C. Pies and M. Heliquist (eds) *Face to Face: a Guide to AIDS Counselling*, AIDS Health Project, University of California, San Francisco, California.

Gallia, K.S. (1996) Teaching spiritual care: beyond content. *Nursing Connections*, **9**(3), 29–35.

George, H. (1989) Counselling people with AIDS, their lovers, friends and relations. In: J. Green, and A. McCreaner, (eds) *Counselling in HIV Infection and AIDS*, Blackwell, London.

Gostin, L.O. (1990) The AIDS Litigation Project: a national review of court and human rights commission decisions. Part II: Discrimination. *Journal of the American Medical Association*, **263**, 2086–93.

Green, J. and Davey, T. (1992) Counselling with the 'worried well'. *Counselling Psychology Quarterly*, **5**(2), 213–20.

Hall, C. (1954) *A Primer of Freudian Psychology*, Mentor Books, New York.

Halmos, P. (1965) *The Faith of the Counsellors*, Constable, London.

Harris, T. (1969) *I'm OK, You're OK*, Harper and Row, London.

Haydn, H. (1965) Humanism in 1984. *American Scholar*, **35**, 12–27.

Hayward, J. (1975) *Informative: a Prescription Against Pain*, Royal College of Nursing, London.

Hein, K. (1989) Commentary on adolescent acquired immunodeficiency syndrome: the next wave of the human immunodeficiency virus epidemic? *Journal of Pediatrics*, **114**, 144–9.

Henggeler, S. W., Melton, G.B. and Rodrigue, J.R. (1992) *Pediatric and Adolescent AIDS: Research Findings from the Social Sciences*, Sage, Newbury Park, California.

Herbert, J.T. (1996) Use of adventure-based counselling programs for persons with disabilities. *Journal of Rehabilitation*, **62**(4), 3–9.

Heron, J. (1970) *The Phenomenology of the Gaze*, Human Potential Research Project, University of Surrey, Guildford, Surrey.

Heron, J. (1973) *Experiential Training Techniques*, Human Potential Research Project, University of Surrey, Guildford, Surrey.

Heron, J. (1977a) *Catharsis in Human Development*, Human Potential Research Project, University of Surrey, Guildford, Surrey.

Heron, J. (1977b) *Behaviour Analysis in Education and Training*, Human Potential Research Project, University of Surrey, Guildford, Surrey.

Heron, J. (1978) *Co-Counselling Teacher's Manual*, Human Potential Research Project, University of Surrey, Guildford, Surrey.

Heron, J. (1981) Philosophical basis for a new paradigm. In: P. Reason and J. Rowan (eds) *Human Inquiry: a Sourcebook of new Paradigm Research*, Wiley, Chichester.

Heron, J. (1986) *Six Category Intervention Analysis*, 2nd edn, Human Potential Research Project, University of Surrey, Guildford, Surrey.

Heron, J. (1989) *Helping the Client*, Sage, London.

Hesse, H. (1927) *Steppenwolf*, Penguin, Harmondsworth.
Hesse, H. (1979) *My Belief*, Panther, St Albans.
Hobbs, T. (1992) Skills in communication and counselling. In: T. Hobbs (ed.) *Experiential Training: Practical Guidelines*, Routledge, London.
Homans, G.C. (1961) *Social Behavior in its Elementary Forms*, Harcourt Vrace, New York.
Hopkins, G.M. (1953) *Poems and Prose* (ed. W.H. Gardner), Penguin, Harmondsworth.
Hopper, L., Jesson, A. and Macleod Clark, J. (1991) Progression to counselling. *Nursing Times*, 87(8), 41–3.
Hopson, B. (1985) Adult life and career counselling. *British Journal of Guidance and Counselling*, **13**(1), 49–59.
Howard, A. (1990) Counselling PLC. *Counselling: The Journal of the British Association for Counselling*, **1**(1), 15–16.
Howard, G.S., Nance, D.W. and Myers, P. (1987) *Adaptive Counselling and Therapy: a Systematic Approach to Selecting Effective Treatments*, Jossey-Bass, San Francisco.
Howe, J. (1989) AIDS – The rights approach. *Professional Nurse*, **5**(3), 156–9.
Hurt, R.D., Dale, L.C., Fredrickson, P.A., *et al.* (1994) Nicotine patch therapy for smoking cessation combined with physician advice and nurse follow up: one-year outcome and percentage of nicotine replacement. *Journal of the American Medical Association*, **271**(8), 595–600.
Hurtig, W. and Fandrick, C. (1990) The nursing student and the psychiatric patient with AIDS: a case study. *Nurse Education Today* **10**(2), 92–7.
Jackins, H. (1965) *The Human Side of Human Beings*, Rational Island Publishers, Seattle, Washington.
Jackins, H. (1970) *Fundamentals of Co-Counselling Manual*, Rational Island Publishers, Seattle, Washington.
Jackson, P.L. and Vessey, J.A. (1992) *Primary Care of the Child with a Chronic Condition*, Mosby Year Book, St Louis.
James, M. and Jongeward, D. (1971) *Born to Win: Transactional Analysis with Gestalt Experiments*, Addison-Wesley, Reading, Mass.
James, W. (1890) *The Principles of Psychology*, Henry Holt, New York.
Jerrett, M. and Evans, K. (1986) Children's pain vocabulary. *Journal of Advanced Nursing*, **11**, 403–8.
Jourard, S. (1964) *The Transparent Self*, Van Nostrand, Princeton, New Jersey.
Jung, C.G. (1978) Selected Writings, Fontana, London.
Kagan, C., Evans, J. and Kay, B. (1986) *A Manual of Interpersonal Skills for Nurses: an Experiential Approach*, Harper and Row, London.
Kahn, R.L. and Cannell, C.F. (1957) *The Dynamics of Interviewing*, Wiley, New York.
Kalisch, B.J. (1971) Strategies for developing nurse empathy. *Nursing Outlook*, **19**(11), 714–17.
Kelly, G. (1955) *The Psychology of Personal Constructs*, Vols 1 and 2, Norton, New York.
Kelly, G. (1963) The autobiography of a theory. In: D. Bannister and J.M.M. Mair (eds) *The Evaluation of Personal Construct Theory*, Academic Press, London.
Kirschenbaum, R. (1978) *On Becoming Carl Rogers*, Dell, New York.
Kolb, D. (1984) *Experiential Learning*, Prentice-Hall, Englewood Cliffs, New Jersey.

Kopp, S. (1974) *If You Meet the Buddha on the Road, Kill Him!: A Modern Pilgrimage Through Myth, Legend and Psychotherapy*, Sheldon Press, London.

Lago, C. and Thompson, J. (1989) Counselling and race. In: W. Dryden, D. Charles-Edwards and R. Woolfe (eds.) *Handbook of Counselling in Britain*, Routledge, London.

Laing, R.D. (1959) *The Divided Self*, Penguin, Harmondsworth.

Langer, N. (1997) Training for retirement counselling in a Master of Arts in social gerontology curriculum. *Gerontology and Geriatrics Education*, **18**(2), 87–95.

Langley, T. (1995) Training staff to provide a continence helpline. *Professional Nurse*, **11**(2), 121–4.

Lansdown, R. (1992) Coping with child death: a child's view. *Nursing*, **2**(43), 1263–6.

Leininger, L.S. and Earp, J.A.L. (1993) The effect of training staff in office-based smoking cessation. *Patient Education and Counselling*, **20**(1), 17–25.

Leukefeld, C.G. (1988) AIDS counselling and testing. *Health and Social Work*, **13**(3) 167–9.

Lewis, H. and Streitfield, H. (1971) *Growth Games*, Bantam Books, New York.

Licavoli, L. and Hahn, N.I. (1995) Dietetics goes into therapy: nutrition therapists replace rules with understanding. *Journal of the American Dietetic Association*, **95**(7), 751–2.

Lourea, D.N. (1985) Psychosocial issues related to counselling bisexuals. *Journal of Homosexuality*, **11**(1–2), 52–62.

Lowen, A. (1967) *Betrayal of the Body*, Macmillan, New York.

Lowen, A. and Lowen, L. (1977) *The Way to Vibrant Health: a Manual of Bioenergetic Exercises*, Harper and Row, New York.

Luft, J. (1969) *Of Human Interaction: the Johari Model*, Mayfield, Palo Alto, California.

MacCaffrey, E.A. (1987) Counselling AIDS patients: a unique approach by Shanti therapists. *AIDS Patient Care* **1**(2), 26–7.

Macleod Clark, J., Hopper, L. and Jesson, A. (1991) Progression to counselling, *Nursing Times*, **87**(8), 41–3.

Macquarrie, J. (1973) *Existentialism*, Penguin, Harmondsworth.

Masson, J. (1990) *Against Therapy*, Fontana, London.

Masson, J. (1992) *Final Analysis: the Making and Unmaking of a Psychoanalyst*, Fontana, London.

May, R. (1983) *The Discovery of Being*, Norton, New York.

Mayeroff, M. (1972) *On Caring*, Harper and Row, New York.

McClain, M. and Mandell, F. (1994) Sudden infant death syndrome: the nurse counselor's response to bereavement counselling, *Journal of Community Health Nursing*, **11**(3), 177–86.

McCreaner, A. (1989) Pre-test counselling. In: J. Green and A. McCreaner, (eds) *Counselling in HIV Infection and AIDS*, Blackwell, London.

McGough, K.N. (1990) Assessing social support for people with AIDS. *Oncology Nursing Forum*, **17**(1), 31–5.

McLaren, M.C. (1998) *Interpreting Cultural Differences: the Challenge of Intercultural Communication*, Peter Francis, Norfolk.

McLeod, J. (1993) *Introduction to Counselling*, Open University Press, Buckingham.

McLeod, J. (1998) *An Introduction to Counselling*, 2nd edn, Open University Press, Buckingham.

Mehrabian, D. (1971) *Silent Messages*, Wadsworth, Belmont, California.

MGC (1983) *Aims, Beliefs and Organisation*, National Marriage Guidance Council, Rugby.

Miller, C. (1990) *The AIDS Handbook*, Penguin, Harmondsworth.

Miller, D. (1987) *Living with AIDS and HIV*, Macmillan, London.

Miller, R. (1995) Suicide and AIDS: problem identification during counselling. *AIDS Care*, 7(supplement 2), 199–205.

Miller, R. and Bor, R. (1990) *Counselling for HIV screening in women*. In: Studd, J. (ed.) *Progress in Obstetrics and Gynaecology*, Churchill Livingstone, Edinburgh.

Miller, R., Goldman, E., Bor, R. *et al.* (1989) Counselling children and adults about AIDS/HIV. *Counselling Psychology Quarterly*, 2, 65–72.

Morris, D. (1978) *Manwatching: a Field Guide to Human Behaviour*, Triad/Panther, St Albans.

Morrison, P. and Burnard, P. (1997) *Caring and Communicating: the Interpersonal Relationship in Nursing*, 2nd edn, Macmillan, Basingstoke.

Moskowitz, E. and Jennings, B. (1996) Public health policy forum. Directive counselling on long-acting contraception. *American Journal of Public Health*, **86**(6), 787–90.

Mullins, J., Roessler, R., Schriner, K., Brown, P. and Bellini, J. (1997) Improving employment outcomes through quality rehabilitation. *Journal of Rehabilitation*, **63**(4), 21–31.

Munro, A., Manthei, B. and Small, J. (1989) *Counselling: Skills of Problem Solving*, Routledge, London.

Murgatroyd, S. (1986) *Counselling and Helping*, British Psychological Society and Methuen, London.

Murgatroyd, S. and Woolfe, R. (1982) *Coping with Crisis: Understanding and Helping Persons in Need*, Harper and Row, London.

Murphy, G. and Kovach, J.K. (1972) *Historical Introduction to Modern Psychology*, 6th edn, Routledge and Kegan Paul, London.

Myerscough, P.R. (1989) *Talking With Patients*, Oxford Medical Publications, Oxford.

Nelson-Jones, R. (1995) *The Theory and Practice of Counselling*, Cassell, London.

O'Connor, F. (1998) Good country people. In: R. Ford (ed.) *The Granta Book of the American Short Story*, Granta, London.

O'Driscoll, M. (1997) Let's talk about sex: providing both sex education and sexual health education to young people. *Nursing Times*, **93**(49), 34–5.

Off Pink Collective (1988) *Bisexual Lives*, Off Pink Collective, London.

Ornstein, R.E. (1975) *The Psychology of Consciousness*, Penguin, Harmondsworth.

Pakta, F. (ed.) (1972) *Existential Thinkers and Thought*, Citadel Press, Secaucus, New Jersey.

Parkinson, F. (1993) *Post-Trauma Stress*, Sheldon Press, London.

Patton, M.Q. (1982) *Practical Evaluation*, Sage, Beverly Hills, California.

Pearce, B. (1989) Counselling skills in the context of professional and organizational growth. In: W. Dryden, D. Charles-Edwards and R. Woolfe (eds) *Handbook of Counselling in Britain*, Routledge, London.

Perls, F. (1969) *Gestalt Therapy Verbatim*, Real People Press, Lafayette, California.

Perls, F., Hefferline, R.F. and Goodman, P. (1951) *Gestalt Therapy: Excitement and Growth in the Human Personality*, Penguin, Harmondsworth.

Pfeiffer, J.W. and Jones, J.E. (1974) *A Handbook of Structured Exercises for Human Relations Training*, University Associates, La Jolla, California.

Polanyi, M. (1958) *Personal Knowledge*, University of Chicago Press, Chicago.

Pring, R. (1976) *Knowledge and Schooling*, Open Books, London.

Prosser, G. (1985) Communication as social interaction. In: A. Braithwaite and D. Rogers, (eds) *Children Growing Up*, Open University Press, Milton Keynes.

Reich, W. (1949) *Character Analysis*, Simon and Schuster, New York.

Riebel, L. (1984) A homeopathic model of psychotherapy. *Journal of Humanistic Psychology*, **24**(1), 9–48.

Rogers, C.R. (1951) *Client-Centred Therapy*, Constable, London.

Rogers, C.R. (1957) The necessary and sufficient conditions of therapuetic personality change. *Journal of Consulting Psychology*, **21**, 95–104.

Rogers, C.R. (1967) *On Becoming a Person: a Therapist's View of Psychotherapy*, Constable, London.

Rogers, C.R. (1983) *Freedom to Learn for the Eighties*, Merrill, Columbus, Ohio.

Rogers, C.R. (1985) Toward a more human science of the person. *Journal of Humanistic Psychology*, **25**(4), 7–24.

Rogers, C.R. and Dymond, R.F. (1978) *Psychotherapy and Personality Change*, University of Chicago Press, Chicago.

Rogers, C.R. and Stevens, B. (1967) *Person to Person: the Problem of Being Human*, Real People Press, Lafayette, California.

Ross, L.A. (1996) Teaching spiritual care to nurses. *Nurse Education Today*, **16**(1), 38–43.

Rowe, D. (1987) Introduction. In: J. Masson (ed.) *Against Therapy*, Fontana, London.

Ryle, G. (1949) *The Concept of Mind*, Penguin, Harmondsworth.

Sartre, J.-P. (1956) *Being and Nothingness*, Philosophical Library, New York.

Sartre, J.-P. (1965) *Nausea*, Penguin, Harmondsworth.

Sartre, J.-P. (1973) *Existentialism and Humanism*, Methuen, London.

Schulman, D. (1982) *Intervention in Human Services: a Guide to Skills and Knowledge*, 3rd edn, C.V. Mosby, St Louis, Missouri.

Searle, J.R. (1983) *Intentionality: an Essay in Philosophy of the Mind*, Cambridge University Press, Cambridge.

Sennott-Miller, L. and Kligman, E. W. (1992) Healthier lifestyles: how to motivate older patients to change. *Geriatrics*, **47**(12), 52–9.

Shaffer, J.B.P. (1978) *Humanistic Psychology*, Prentice-Hall, Englewood Cliffs, New Jersey.

Shapiro, L. (1984) *The New Short-term Therapies for Children: a Guide for the Helping Professions and Parents*, Prentice-Hall, New Jersey.

Simon, S.B., Howe, L.W. and Kirschenbaum, H. (1978) *Values Clarification*, revised edition, A and W Visual Library, New York.

Sketchley, J. (1989) Counselling people affected by HIV and AIDS. In: W. Dryden, D. Charles-Edwards and R. Woolfe (eds) *Handbook of Counselling in Britain*, Routledge, London.

Smith, C.E., Haynes, K., Rebeck, S.L. *et al.* (1998) Patients as peer preceptors for orthopedic oncology rehabilitation patients. *Rehabilitation Nursing*, **23**(2), 78–83.

Smith, E.W.L. (ed.) (1976) *The Growing Edge of Gestalt Therapy*, Citadel Press, Secaucus, New Jersey.

Stedeford, A. (1989) Counselling, death and bereavement. In: W. Dryden, D. Charles-Edwards and R. Woolfe, (eds) *Handbook of Counselling in Britain*, Routledge, London.

Steil, L. (1991) Listening training: the key to success in today's organisations. In: D. Borisoff and M. Purdy (eds) *Listening in Everyday Life*, University of America Press, Maryland.

Stewart, V. and Stewart, A. (1981) *Business Applications of Repertory Grid*, McGraw Hill, London.
Storr, A. (ed.) (1983) *Jung: Selected Writings*, Fontana, London.
Street, E. (1989) Family counselling. In: W. Dryden, D. Charles-Edwards and R. Woolfe (eds) *Handbook of Counselling in Britain*, Routledge, London.
Tennen, H., Rohrbaugh, M., Press, S. and White, L. (1981) Reactance theory and therapeutic paradox: a compliance-defiance model. *Psychotherapy: Theory, Research and Practice)*, 18(1), 14–22.
Theroux, P. (1977) *The Great Railway Bazaar*, Penguin, Harmondsworth.
Tillich, P. (1952) *The Courage to Be*, Yale University Press, New Haven, Connecticut.
Truax, C.B. and Carkuff, R.R. (1967) *Towards Effective Counselling and Psychotherapy*, Aldine, Chicago.
Tschudin, V. (1991) *Counselling Skills for Nurses*, Baillière Tindall, London.
Vonnegut, K. (1968) *Mother Night*, Cape, London.
Wallis, R. (1984) *Elementary Forms of the New Religious Life*, Routledge and Kegan Paul, London.
Watkins, J. (1978) *The Therapeutic Self*, Human Science Press, New York.
Wheeler, D.D. and Janis, I.L. (1980) *A Practical Guide for Making Decisions*, Free Press, New York.
Wilkinson, J. and Canter, S. (1982) *Social Skills Training Manual: Assessement, Programme Design and Management of Training*, Wiley, Chichester.
Williams, D. (1997) *Communication Skills in Practice: a Practical Guide for Health Professionals*, Jessica Kingsley, London.
Wilson, C. (1955) *The Outsider*, Gollancz, London.
Winbolt, B. (1997) Just words away from harm: counselling and the breaking of bad news. *Therapy Weekly*, 23(26), 6.
Youll, J. and Wilson, K. (1996) A therapeutic approach to bereavement counselling. *Nursing Times*, 92(16), 40–2.

Index